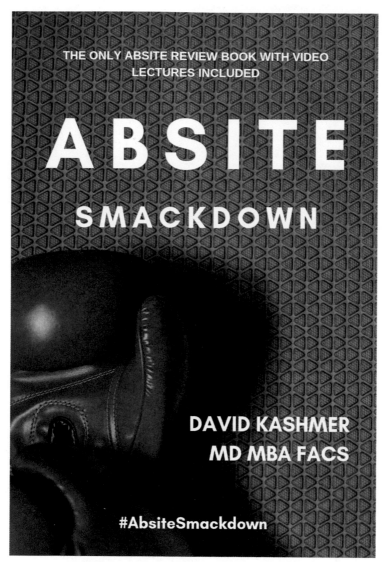

THE ONLY ABSITE REVIEW BOOK WITH VIDEO LECTURES INCLUDED

ABSITE

SMACKDOWN

DAVID KASHMER
MD MBA FACS

#AbsiteSmackdown

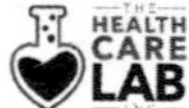

THE HEALTHCARE LAB, INC.

ABSITE Smackdown!

The Absite Review Manual With Video Review Course

David Kashmer, MD MBA

 This work is based on the *ABSITE: Smackdown* video lecture series, multiple content sources (including, but not limited to, surgeons' notes), and expert opinion. This work is meant to enable content review in preparation for the ABSITE and is **not** meant to guide or direct the care of patients. This is not a guide on how to practice the Art and Science of Surgery. As a result, the publisher will not be liable for error, omission, inaccuracy or for any damage that results from applying this work in the care of patients.

Table Of Contents

Why I Wrote This Book

My intern year was a tough one: new place, long hours, and a *whole* lot of other new experiences.

One of them was the ABSITE exam.

I didn't know (until too late) that the ABSITE was given in January every year. Just too busy working I guess.

I *definitely* didn't think to try and make sure I wasn't on call the night *before* the ABSITE. That would've needed to be done months ahead of time.

When I did wind up on call, I didn't have a great plan for how to get through the test the next day.

Perhaps predictably, that first ABSITE didn't go so well for me.

A lack of sleep, lack of understanding about key performance factors, and a weak knowledge base did NOT make for a good performance. Like with most things, some of the root causes were modifiable and some were not.

It's a good policy, I think, to focus on the factors we can control. Especially when we perform poorly.

Otherwise, we never learn what we could've done better and think we are blameless.

At the same time, there are some things we can't really influence. So we focus on what we can improve.

Afterward, I made it my business to eliminate all the barriers I could to improving my performance on the ABSITE.

I looked for the right books, right understanding of the test, and right preparation for what was coming each January.

Now, these many years after residency and subsequent fellowships, I want to share with you the resources I've shared with residents for more than ten years about current content tested on the ABSITE, the nature of the test, and how to make sure you perform the best you can on that yearly assessment.

Unlike every other review book I've ever seen, this one comes with a video review course built right in.

ABSITE: Smackdown!

Instructions on how to access your video review course are included here in your book. Just check out the later section on *How To Unlock Your Video Review Course*—remember, it's easy: it just takes an email with your proof of purchase for this book! When you purchased this book you purchased that review course already.

The course is based on the same content in the book, and has a lot of great photos and additional content. It's portable, which was *very* important to me (and the publishers) so that it allows you to have it on hand anytime you have your phone, tablet, or computer. Each section has an associated lecture.

No need to fly anywhere for an ABSITE review course if you can help it. And with this one, you can watch or listen to it while you eat or whenever it's comfortable! (Coffee, pajamas, and an ABSITE video review course...what could be better?) Not to mention, those review courses typically cost $595 AND a plane ticket...and don't forget about your travel time!

Until now, these barriers prevented many residents from taking a course at all.

So I looked for a way to save busy surgery residents money AND get them both a book and review course especially for the ABSITE...because I remember how tight funds can be when you're a resident. Thanks to the publisher, this book and course generally makes things much easier.

By supporting the course and buying this book, you're helping the team constantly improve the work along with that accompanying review course!

Anyhow, even if the ABSITE gave me an early smackdown, I definitely returned the favor to that exam for years afterward and share this to help continue the trend.

With this work, I want to help you to deliver that same smackdown to the ABSITE...whether this is your first or final year taking that test.

Take a look inside to learn the tools, test content, and some techniques to dropkick the ABSITE into next year.

And by the way: again, this ABSITE book is different. In addition to arming you with the content you need for the test, I wanted to share with you those key factors for performance on the test along with that great video review course to have on hand anytime and anywhere.

Good luck, and remember to share this work with friends and colleagues so we can go on improving the book and course to help them for years to come!

Why You Should Read This Book

It may be June, it may be January...no matter. This book will help you perform your best on the ABSITE.

I've read more than 15 ABSITE review books so that you don't have to.

And more importantly, I've included key factors (besides just content) that help you perform on the ABSITE along with an entire video review course based on the content here.

Now hear this: will ONE review book cover everything you need for the ABSITE?

No way.

Although this book and course cover similar content to many other reviews, no one review book (or course) covers *everything* you need for the test. Trust me, to claim otherwise is foolish.

This book, however, covers useful ABSITE content and adds those additional performance tips that others do not. It's as much of one-stop-shopping for you as I've ever seen along with some useful extras.

In this book, I'll share some evidence about performance on the ABSITE that can help drive you to your best score.

I'll tell you specifics about how the ABSITE is given, how many questions there are, and what the sources are for the content in those questions.

I'll also share the content that is frequently tested on the ABSITE in an easy to read, quick format.

Maybe most importantly, this book is alive and is frequently updated based on your feedback. It's constantly improving.

At the end of the book, I'll share a quick link for you to give your feedback about the book (and the video course) to improve things for future generations of test takers.

This book is worth your precious time—it won't take much of it, but it *will* deliver lots of useful help to make sure you demonstrate your surgical knowledge to the best of your ability on that yearly assessment called the ABSITE.

It will also teach you specific factors that help you perform your best this time around.

Now let's get to it!

Facts About The ABSITE

Once upon a time, the ABSITE was administered as *one* test...and on paper!

Then things changed. In an effort to recognize differences between senior and junior residents, the American Board of Surgery, keepers of the American Board of Surgery Inservice Training Exam (ABSITE), created a senior and junior version of the test for administration each year.

And then things changed again!

In 2014, the ABSITE returned to the single-test format. Now, all surgery residents take one version of the test meant for all year levels.

The test is administered on computers. It is administered by each residency program as a single five hour block.

There are approximately 250 multiple choice questions on the test. The test is administered in January and your residency program receives your results in March along with other score reports about the residency's performance.

Just so you know, the ABSITE is NOT required for eventual board certification in Surgery...but I've never heard or seen an accredited residency program that did not use the ABSITE every year.

Residency programs must order the ABSITE materials from the American Board of Surgery (ABS), and the residency program is responsible for administering the test to residents. Residencies do pay the ABS for the exam materials.

The ABS will *not* send you any information directly about your ABSITE. Everything you want to know must come from your program. If you call or write the ABS to discuss something about your test, you'll be referred right back to your program.

Your program will typically share your score report with you in March or later.

The ABS looks for certain testing irregularities too. If they feel that something is amiss with the testing process and / or results from your center, they will notify your program director, your Chair of Surgery, and other staff at your institution. They will request an investigation by your program director.

Your program director will choose disciplinary action based on his/her findings. And your program may be severely penalized.

Bottom line: as usual, don't cheat. It's a bad idea.

Also, you can't share questions from the ABSITE with anyone without violating the *ABS Ethics and Professionalism Policy.*

Again, it's a better idea to study and practice than it is to cheat or help someone cheat in any way.

Now that we have all of that out of the way, let me share with you some great resources to understand the format of the test, the content it's based on, and even a useful practice test.

First, here is an important information page and fact sheet all about the ABSITE from the American Board of Surgery. It has much of the information I've shared with you earlier.

Before you dive into the factual content in the rest of the book, take a look at this page by clicking on the link. If the link doesn't open or you're reading in paperback, break out your computer and open this address on your web browser:

http://bit.ly/ABSITEinfo

That will bring you to the ABS info page on the ABSITE. Take a look before you start studying facts that will be tested on the ABSITE itself.

Don't worry...when these webpages eventually move or change location, the book will be updated so that the links shared here still work!

Next up, here's a link directly to ABSITE content sheet from the ABS:

http://bit.ly/ABSITEcontent

Basically, it shares some important facts about current ABSITE content, including:

- ABSITE follows the Surgical Council on Resident Education (SCORE) curriculum
- 80% of the ABSITE focuses on Clinical Management topics, and 20% covers Applied Science (used to be called "Basic Science") topics
- 72% of the questions concern SCORE Patient Care topics, 24% SCORE Medical Knowledge topics, and 4% are about "other" topics

That content sheet is great because it even shares specific categories and how much they are focused on in the test. Take a look at PDF from that link, page 2, for sure before you study.

Once you've looked at the link about ABSITE info and ABSITE content (along with weighting) this useful link on the SCORE curriculum will tell you what each of those content areas mean:

http://bit.ly/ABSoutline

And with that you've looked at what the ABSITE is, what it covers, how it's weighted, and what, specifically, each content area means.

Before we get into the specifics about what's tested, and all the interesting facts we know and love that are tested on the ABSITE, it's also worthwhile to get to know how the test interface works on the computer. Here's a practice test interface for you:

http://bit.ly/ABSITEpractice

With that, you've learned about how the test looks, what's covered, and how long the test typically is.

By the way...before we move along: review books are *great*—especially when you don't have time or ability to review the complete book or work.

However, review books like this one don't substitute for things like the full SCORE curriculum. Working and studying over time promotes long term retention. This book will help you, and it doesn't substitute for long term study with SCORE and other works.

Now let's get some facts about whether the ABSITE predicts eventual success on passing your board exam...

Summary

- The ABSITE is now one test version that is given to all PGY levels.
- It is administered by each residency program as a single 5 hour block. There are approximately 250 multiple choice questions on the test. The test is administered in January.
- DON'T CHEAT on the test. The obvious reason is because cheating prevents the test from functioning as an indicator of what you know. Another important reason is that your program (and you) will have a *host* of problems if the ABS thinks there may be "testing irregularities".
- ABSITE follows the SCORE curriculum.
- These links are incredibly useful to teach you what content will be tested, how it lines up with SCORE, specifics about what SCORE for each section includes, and how the computer testing interface looks and feels:
    - http://bit.ly/ABSITEinfo
    - http://bit.ly/ABSITEcontent
    - http://bit.ly/ABSoutline
    - http://bit.ly/ABSITEpractice
- Review books like this one don't substitute for things like the full SCORE curriculum. Yes, *ABSITE Smackdown* will help you, but it doesn't substitute for working consistently over time to master surgical content.

Does the ABSITE Predict Success On Boards?

Quick! Click this link and take a look at the abstracts it brings up on Pubmed:

http://bit.ly/ABSITEpredictsboards

So what do you think? Does ABSITE performance predict whether you'll pass boards?

It's sort of a mixed bag, right? On the one hand, scoring less than the 35th percentile correlates with not passing boards. On the other hand, the ABSITE seems to correlate with passing the first portion of the board exam (the qualifying exam) but not the second portion (the certification exam aka "oral boards").

And you know what? It doesn't really matter whether ABSITE correlates with boards or does not. Here's why...

I've sat in many faculty meetings to evaluate residents. You know what often comes up? ABSITE scores. Just like the article in the link above describes, decisions about PGY year promotion, probationary status, and LOTS of other important decisions look to ABSITE scores. After all, the score is a number...so people believe it's pretty concrete.

Is that right? Wrong? Dunno. It just is what it is.

And now hear this: there's even evidence about what factors lead to improvement in ABSITE scores.

http://bit.ly/ABSITEfactorstoimprove

From that study, it sounds like whether you're on probation, how anxious you are about the exam, conference attendance, and several other key factors give improvement in ABSITE score.

I won't comment more here or share my opinion on the findings, but I will share that I'd love to look at some different items that may help explain performance.

For now, just be aware: does the ABSITE predict success on boards? Sort of. But, more importantly, it's used throughout residency to assess your progress and, in some programs, may play into whether you're promoted to the next year.

It was originally designed as a tool to help program directors assess strengths of their educational program and what residents needed; now, like many things, it's taken on a greatly expanded role.

Take it seriously. ABSITE performance will have significant implications on your time in residency.

Summary

- Does the ABSITE predict your ability to pass boards? Sort of. Look here: http://bit.ly/ABSITEpredictsboards
- There's even some evidence about what factors yield improvement in ABSITE scores. http://bit.ly/ABSITEfactorstoimprove
- Does it *matter* whether the ABSITE truly predicts your ability to pass boards? Probably not, because it's used for all sorts of things throughout residency to assess you. It's just plain important.
- The ABSITE was originally designed to help program directors assess their educational programs. It's become much more than that. It's used to help make decisions regarding promotion and probation.

Statistics, Safety, & Decision-Making

Sensitivity: probability that a test is positive in diseased patient ("Positive In Disease", or PID)

- Number of people with disease and positive test result divided by total number that actually have disease as determined by whatever the gold standard test is
- Independent of prevalence
- Sensitive test lets you rule out disease (SNOUT = "sensitive rule out")

Specificity: probability that a test is negative in patients who are healthy ("Negative In Health", or NIH)

- Number of people with no disease and negative test result divided by number without disease as determined by whatever the gold standard test is (true negative)
- Higher specificity means better able to rule in disease because test is likely to be negative in truly healthy people
- Very specific tests let you rule in disease more effectively (SPIN = "SPecific rule IN")
- Independent of prevalence

Predictive value of a test *does* depend on disease prevalence

Positive predictive value: true positive tests divided by the sum of true positive tests and false positives

Is the chance that, with a positive test, the patient truly has the disease

Negative predictive value: true negative tests divided by the sum of true negative tests and false negatives

Is the chance that, with a negative test result, the patient does NOT have the disease

Accuracy of a test: the quantity true positive (TP) results plus true negative (TN) results divided by the quantity true positives results plus true negative results plus false positive results (FP) plus false negative results (FN)

- Written differently, accuracy = (TP +TN) / (TP + TN + FP + FN)
- Written differently: all the test results that were correct divided by all results total

Prospective cohort studies have *non-random* assignment to treatment group

Continuous data = data that can be divided infinitely into smaller parts and still have meaning: eg an hour can be divided into minutes, then seconds, then nanoseconds etc etc.

Discrete data are data that come in chunks, eg red, yellow, green...cannot be divided and continue to have meaning.

Qualitative variables are discrete data such as nominal (names like colors) or ordinal (on a scale like happiness rated 1-10)

ANOVA is a t-test for more than 2 samples of continuous data

Non-parametric statistics are for *qualitative* data ie non-numerical data such as patient's demographic data (nationality etc.)

The chi-squared test may be used to compare two groups to determine whether there is a significant difference in the number with / without some trait, eg to determine whether there is a significant difference in the number of people who have a HGBA1C < 7 among diabetic patients versus non-diabetics.

Kaplan-Meyer curves: estimate survival of sample over time

Relative risk: incidence in people exposed to some factor divided by incidence in people who are not exposed

Power: probability of making the correct conclusion based on statistical test

1 - Probability of type 2 error = power

Larger sample increases power

Prevalence is the number of patients having the disease in the population at any one time, and is higher in diseases that patients may have for a long time

Incidence the number of new diagnoses of disease in a given time period (new ones only)

Null hypothesis: no difference exists

Type I Error: "tampering"

- This is when you think there was a difference between something and something else. You may take action based on that incorrect thought and do something to a system. You tampered with the system because there was no difference and you did something that actually may make the situation worse.
- A slightly more confusing way to say the same thing is that you incorrectly rejected the null hypothesis (null hypothesis says there is no difference). But that's more confusing and is filled with double negatives.

Type II Error: "undercontrolling"

- This is when you thought there was NO difference between two things and so you didn't make any changes. But in reality there WAS a difference and you missed it. So you "undercontrolled" for the problem or issue.
- Perhaps a more confusing way to say this is that you incorrectly accepted the null hypothesis.

Prevent gaps in care (shift changes, transfers, new providers coming on call) from injuring patients with structured handoffs (eg checklists), order sets.

Root cause analysis (often performed with Fishbone aka Ishikawa diagram) used to investigate sentinel event (an unexpected event involving risk of serious injury or actual injury to patients)

The *universal protocol* is the JCAHO protocol to prevent wrong site / wrong patient surgery. It involves: surgical site marking (must be visible after site prep), a preoperative checklist, and a time out immediately before incision.

Carter's rule: say your plan for the patient out loud in the most direct, non-medical terms possible. If it sounds like a bad idea, it's a bad idea. If you don't want to say it out loud, it's also a bad idea.

Summary

- Sensitivity (SN) is chance that test is PID. You can use a very sensitive test to rule out disease. SNOUT.
- Specificity (SP) is chance that test is NIH. You can use a very specific test to SPIN.
- Type 1 error is tampering. (Eg: placing a chest tube when none was needed.) Aka rejecting the null hypothesis incorrectly
- Type 2 error is undercontrolling. (Failing to place a chest tube when one WAS needed.) Aka accepting the null hypothesis incorrectly.
- Continuous data can be divided infinitely and will still make sense. Eg length, time, etc.
- 1 – probability of type 2 error = power
- Prevalence and incidence are VERY different. Diseases that linger a long time give higher prevalence. SN and SP do NOT depend on prevalence, but predictive value of a test does.
- Universal protocol is JCAHO protocol for preventing wrong site / wrong patient surgery and has important elements.

Hepatobiliary

Right hepatic artery comes off SMA in 17%-20% of patients. This "replaced right" is the most common hepatic artery variant. Some question about it comes up very often on the ABSITE.

Replaced left hepatic artery comes off left gastric artery and is found in gastrohepatic ligament. Slightly less commonly seen than replaced right.

Falciform ligament contains remnant of LEFT umbilical vein

Separates parts of left lobe of liver into medial and lateral segments

Ligamentum teres extends from falciform and is remnant of obliterated LEFT umbilical vein. Goes to underside of liver.

Cantile's line is imaginary line drawn from IVC to gallbladder fossa and separates liver into left and right lobes.

Couinaud's segments lined up with left and right lobes:

- Left lobe = segments 2, 3, 4
- Right lobe = 5, 6, 7, 8

Segment 1 is caudate lobe

Gallbladder is under segment 4 & 5 and portal triad enters at segments 4 & 5.

NB: on the test, segments may be written with Roman numerals instead of the typical digits used here. Segment 4 may be written as IV, etc.

Most liver tumors are supplied by hepatic artery. This holds true for primary and metastatic tumors.

Relationship of portal triad structures:

D A
V E

D = common bile duct

A = hepatic artery (only artery in body that has naturally occurring, palpable thrill)

V = portal vein

E = empty

- This diagram is as if you were looking from patient's feet toward patient's head
- Duct is anterior and lateral to vein (toward patient's right)
- Artery is anterior to vein and medial to duct, etc. etc.
- (Btw my name is Dave so this helps me remember)

macrophages in liver = Kupffer cells

Pringle maneuver will NOT stop bleeding from replaced L hepatic artery or (more importantly) hepatic veins or IVC

Pringle maneuver = clamping portal triad (DAVe) in hepatoduodenal ligament

Portal vein is formed when splenic vein joins superior mesenteric vein (SMV). Note inferior mesenteric vein enters splenic vein earlier and does NOT join directly with SMV to form portal vein.

- Portal vein delivers 2/3 of blood flow to liver, but this blood has less 02 content than arterial blood. So even though it delivers 2/3 of flow, it delivers roughly half of the 02 to liver. Hepatic artery delivers other half of 02 and 1/3 of blood flow.
- Left portal vein supplies segments 2, 3, & 4. Right portal supplies 5, 6, 7 & 8. Note that caudate lobe (segment 1) is not included in there.
- no valves in portal system

Hepatorenal syndrome is associated with low urinary Na

Cholangitis is fever, RUQ tenderness, & jaundice

Cholangitis + hypotension & change in mental status = Reynaud's pentad

Needs immediate IV abx, fluid resuscitation and emergent drainage of CBD

T tube cholangiogram with retained CBD stone multiple weeks postop is managed by radiology with stone retrieval

#1 cause of benign biliary stricture is lap chole (therefore iatrogenic)

Note that with gallbladder adenocarcinoma 90% patients also have stones. Cholecystectomy adequate if lesion confined to mucosa.

If grossly visible tumor, do regional lymphadenectomy, wedge resection segment 5, skeletonize portal triad (take nodes).

Porcelain gallbladder is associated with 30-65% risk of cancer. Perform cholecystectomy.

Hemobilia triad = GI bleed, jaundice, RUQ pain. workup (and treat) with arteriogram

Gallbladder concentrates bile by active absorption of Na, Cl (H2O then follows)

Hepatic adenoma: 10% rupture/bleed. Also have malignant potential. Liver scan shows these as cold nodules. Presence of hepatic adenoma is an indication for resection.

Hepatic hemangioma: no resection unless giant or symptomatic/consumptive.

Kasaback Merritt syndrome is consumptive coagulopathy or congestive heart failure due to hemangioma. Sometimes seen in children.

Amebic abscess: treatment is metronidazole and NOT surgical. May have "anchovy paste" appearance.

Initial therapy for amebic liver abscess: medical treatment with goal of eliminating organism from the intestinal tract, liver and abscess through the use of METRONIDAZOLE.

- This agent has replaced chloroquine and emetine. 400 mg of metronidazole TID for 4 days.
- This is combined with percutaneous aspiration of the cyst if necessary.
- Patient not considered for surgical treatment until the intestinal phase controlled.
- Medical therapy should precede aspiration attempts by several days.
- Usually aspiration is not required, and abscess resolves medication.

Hydatid cyst is an echinococcal cyst

- Positive Casoni skin test
- Positive indirect hemagglutination
- resect (pericystectomy)

Hepatocellular CA

- #1 CA worldwide.
- May have high alpha fetoprotein.
- Chronic Hep B and C is #1 cause
- Also associated with cirrhosis from ANY cause
- Fibrolamellar variant has better prognosis

Most liver tumors derive blood supply from hepatic artery.

Factor 8, Von Willebrand's Factor, is NOT made in the liver and is located on the endothelium of blood vessels.

Factor 5 Leyden (factor V leyden) is the ONLY factor made COMPLETELY in the liver. Its levels are sometimes used to determine the function of a transplanted liver because of that fact. Especially in liver recipients who have received FFP post op where INR is no longer reliable.

The ONLY water soluble vitamin stored in the liver is B12.

Otherwise, the liver stores fat soluble vitamins (ADEK)

About ¾ of the liver (by weight) can be safely removed without sacrificing function. (In non-cirrhotic liver obviously.)

Hemoglobin is degraded to heme, biliverdin, and then bilirubin. Bilirubin is conjugated to glucaronic acid by glucoronyl transferase in the liver and then is secreted into bile.

Vinyl Chloride Exposure: Vinyl chloride is a carcinogen. May cause cancer specifically in the lung, **liver** and brain. It is a chemical used in the plastics industry.

Exposure to vinyl chloride has been linked to the development of angiosarcoma of the liver.

Complications related to laparoscopic cholecystectomy

- The quoted mortality is <1% with a morbidity level of around 3%.
- Complications include bleeding, infection, risks associated with a general anesthetic, injury to the biliary tree and surrounding organs, and injury to vascular structures.
- There are risks which are unique to laparoscopic techniques. These include extraperitoneal insufflation, gas embolism and trocar induced injuries.

- Complications classified into two major categories:
  - Intraoperative Complications: Damage to the biliary tree, if recognized intraoperatively, should be repaired primarily if possible. Can be done through the laparoscope or an open conversion depending on the skills of the surgeon and the clinical indications.
    - Indications for conversion include (in the order of decreasing frequency):
      - Inadequate visualization of anatomy secondary to inflammation, bleeding, anomalies, or adhesions.
      - Technical complications due to loss of video may require an open approach.
  - Postoperative Complications:
    - These include early recognition of complications, early repair, proper identification of biliary anatomy prior to undertaking a reoperation, and preoperative catheterization of the ductal system via ERCP if indicated. Diagnosis of injuries or complications should be made early.
    - A high index of suspicion is central. Unusually persistent abdominal pain, pain out of proportion or in unlikely areas, hyperbilirubinemia and signs of cholangitis should prompt the surgeon to search for underlying pathology.
    - In the case of common duct injury, a hepaticojejunostomy should be performed.
    - A HIDA scan or ultrasound of the biliary fossa is useful adjunct in addition to a thorough physical exam and essential blood tests.
      ERCP can be useful for stenting cystic duct leaks or removing retained stones without the need for open surgery. Furthermore, it can also aid in diagnosis of biliary stricture or anastomotic leak.

Treatment of hepatic metastases from colon cancer:

- 50% of patients with gastrointestinal tumors have hepatic metastases on autopsy.
- Reasonably long-term survival without recurrence can be obtained in patients with colon cancer metastatic to liver by resection.
- Primary rectal and Wilms' tumors are also good candidates for liver resection.
- Indications for hepatic resection of metastases are:
  - Control of the primary tumor is accomplished or anticipated
  - There are no systemic metastases or abdominal carcinomatosis
  - The patient will tolerate the operative procedure
  - The extent of hepatic involvement is such that resection and total extirpation of the metastasis is feasible.
- If a hepatic metastasis is discovered during a colon resection and it is resectable without anticipated major blood loss, it should be removed at that time.

- Otherwise, resection should be delayed about two months or more, at which time CT scan and angiography should be carried out to assess resectability.
    - Of the 20% of patients with colorectal cancer having hepatic metastasis, ¼ of these are potentially resectable, and ½ of these are not resection candidates because of other metastases.
    - Long-term survival may not be influenced by the interval between resection of the primary lesion and resection of liver metastases.
    - Resection of metastatic hepatic lesion should include a 1cm margin of normal tissue, and can include resection of up to four metastatic tumors without affecting survival.
    - Five year survival rates of 33% have been achieved for patients with hepatic resections for limited hepatic metastases secondary to colon cancer.
    - In non-resectable cases, palliative debulking procedures may be indicated for control of pain associated with hepatic neoplasm.
    - Dearterialization and radiographically controlled embolization can be beneficial in some cases.

Retained CBD stone

- best treated by endoscopic sphincterotomy (success rate 90%, mortality is 1.0-1.5%).
- Extraction of stones > than 1.5 cm. in diameter is seldom possible
- In Billroth II reconstruction, and in distal common duct stricture, surgical approach may be necessary
- Contraindications to endoscopic stone removal:
    - duodenal diverticula, coagulation disorders, and recent pancreatitis.
    - Extracorporeal shock wave lithotripsy is option when stones are too large to extract via the endoscopic approach.
    - If stones are noted on T-tube cholangiogram following a CBD exploration, 5 general approaches are possible (with a T-tube in place and a mature tract):
        - Small stones may be watched since the majority will remain asymptomatic and if not, then may be surgically extracted.
        - Flushing or chemical dissolution (Capmul 8210).
        - Mechanical extraction under x-ray control (using Dormia basket, 90- 96% success).
        - Endoscopic retrieval with transduodenal papillotomy, if the T-tube approach is unsuccessful.
        - Operative intervention.
- success rate for clearance of the duct when multiple stones are present is low when performed by endoscopy. In these situations, choledocholithotomy with choledochoduodenostomy is the procedure of choice.

Anatomy of gallbladder

- no submucosa.
- mucosa is composed of columnar epithelium specialized for absorption of H_2O with concentration of bile.
- Rokitansky–Aschoff sinuses develop from the epithelium through the fibromuscular layer as a result of inflammation and increased intraluminal pressure in the gallbladder. Conditions which cause this include cholecystitis.

Characteristics of cholesterol in bile

- predominately synthesized in the liver.
- rate of synthesis in the liver is regulated through a negative feedback system. (Total body cholesterol synthesis is inhibited by high cholesterol intake.)
- Dietary cholesterol provides an insignificant amount to the overall bile pool.
- Cholesterol gallstones comprise approximately 70% of all gallstones.
- Maintenance of cholesterol in solution is dependent upon sufficient amounts of bile salts and phospholipids.
- Alterations in this balance result in a relative increase in the concentration of cholesterol and may result in the precipitation of cholesterol as stones.
- major vehicle for transport and maintenance of cholesterol in solution are micelles
  - account for approximately 30% of the biliary cholesterol transport. Remainder is carried in a vesicular form.
  - vesicles have lipid bilayers similar to cell membranes.
- precipitation of cholesterol, which may eventually form stones, is in part regulated by glycoproteins found within the mucous secreted in the gallbladder.

Characteristics of cholecystokinin

- Cholecystokinin (CCK) is a 33 amino acid peptide secreted from the duodenum and proximal small intestine.
- Primary Actions:
    - Gallbladder contraction
    - Relaxation of sphincter of Oddi
    - Stimulation of pancreatic secretin
    - Increased intestinal motility
- Secondary Actions (Not Proven):
    - Inhibition of gastric emptying
    - Inhibition of gastric secretion
    - Regulation of pancreatic growth
    - Regulation of satiety
- stimulation of CCK secretion is produced mainly by the presence of fat within the duodenal lumen. ONLY long chain fatty acids (>9 carbon bonds) dispersed in micelles will exert this effect.
- Glucose, aminoacids and other nutrients also stimulate secretion but to a lesser degree.
- several active forms of CCK exist but the 33 and 8 forms are the most active.
- Basal levels of CCK low but increase 5-10 fold with meal ingestion.
- Trypsin is a major regulator of CCK
- Trypsin actively cleaves CCK and renders it **inactive**.
- insulin potentiates CCK, & glucagon inhibits.
- CCK binding results in activation of phospholipase C.
- In this second messenger pathway, ITP-3 and DAG are formed resulting in the intracellular increase of free calcium.
- Calcium binds to calmodulin and then activates indirectly protein kinases responsible for cellular function, namely, pancreatic secretion and synthesis of enzymes.

Characteristics of hepatocytes

- The liver is comprised of three major cell types
    - Kupffer cells (aka macrophages), endothelial lining cells and hepatocytes.
    - Kupffer cells are part of the reticuloendothelial system of the liver that clears antigens via phagocytosis
- Hepatocytes comprise approximately 50% of the total number of cells & make up 80% of the total liver volume.
- Hepatocytes perform most of the metabolic and excretory functions of the liver.
    - Arranged in one cell layered cords called plates.
    - Function depends on their proximity to the hepatic blood supply.
- The hepatocytes can be divided into three major zones:
    - Zone I cells lie in closest proximity to the periportal region and are the first to be exposed to incoming substrates.
        - They are the most susceptible to ischemic insult.
        - So they contain the greatest amount of enzymes and protein substrates. They also produce the majority of proteins and are the main cells responsible for protein metabolism.
- Zone III cells are the farthest away from the oxygen rich blood supply and so they perform glycogenolysis and lipogenesis.
- Ureagenesis occurs in zones II and III.
- Gluconeogenesis occurs in greatest concentration in the proximal periportal area (Zone 1).
- As blood moves from portal to central regions, substrates and metabolites are extracted and added to the blood accordingly.
- Hepatocytes regenerate extremely effectively and rapidly. Estimated that the entire liver mass can be replaced every 50 days.
- This explains the rapid growth of the hepatic remnant after major liver resections. A lot of phosphate is used during this process given the ATP production and cell growth rate involved.

Decreased chloride levels in increased pancreatic exocrine secretion

- The principal cations (positive charged ions) of pancreatic "juice" are sodium and potassium, which are always present in concentrations similar to those found in plasma (the sum of the two is approximately 165 mmol/L).
- The concentration of the principal anions (negative ions), bicarbonate and chloride, varies.
- When there are minimal stimuli to secrete, chloride concentration is high (e.g. 110 mmol/L) and bicarbonate is low, around 50 mmol/L.
- When there is more secretory stimulus, the bicarbonate concentration rises to around 140 mmol/L, and the chloride concentration falls to 20 mmol/L.
- The relationship of the two anions is a result of the passive exchange of intraductal bicarbonate for interstitial chloride.
- Exchange between the two occurs as the juice flows through the larger pancreatic ducts on its way to the duodenum.
- Slower rates give more opportunity for exchange to take place and more for bicarbonate to be lost.
- Alkaline pancreatic juice helps to neutralize gastric acid in the duodenum, thus providing the optimum pH for the activity of pancreatic digestive enzymes.

Jaundice is first seen under the tongue and first appears when total bilirubin is > 2.5

Gilbert's disease: conjugation abnormality with defect in glucuronyl transferase

Crigler-Najjar: inability to conjugate; glucuronyl transferase deficiency

Small Bowel

Gut appears during gestation week 4.

The duodenum: from the junction of the foregut and midgut with recanalization.

The jejunum and proximal portion of the ileum: from proximal limb of the midgut loop

Distal ileum: from caudal limb of the midgut loop.

At week 11 midgut loop rotates 270 degrees counterclockwise around superior mesenteric artery (SMA)

Mucosa includes epithelium, muscularis mucosa, and lamina propria (connective tissue).

Submucosa includes blood vessels, lymphatics, and myenteric Meissner's plexus.

Brunner's glands

at duodenum produce alkaline secretion that protects against acidic gastric chyme.

Lymph aggregates called Peyer's patches are most prevalent in ileum.

Muscularis: Inner circular and outer longitudinal layers. Include myenteric Auerbach's plexus between them.

Serosa: Single layer of mesoepithelial cells which line the exterior of the SI.

Duodenum is first 20 cm of the small bowel.

After ligament of Treitz (LOT) duodenum becomes jejunum. No particular anatomic boundary.

In subsequent 5 or 6 m of small intestine, approximately the proximal 40% is jejunum and distal 60% is ileum.

No anatomic boundaries are present, but the jejunum is differentiated from the ileum by

- greater circumference of jejunum
- longer vasa recta with fewer (1–2) arcades (jejunum)
- plica circulares that are both greater in number and longer (in jejunum)

Enterocytes: Specialize in absorption of dietary nutrients as well as digestion. Greater than 90% of epithelial cells are enterocytes. These arise within crypts of Lieberkühn. They migrate to the villi tips.

Glutamine is preferred fuel of small bowel enterocyte. It is a conditionally essential amino acid (becomes an essential amino acid during stress as body is unable to manufacture it)

Paneth cells: found at the base of the crypts of Lieberkühn. Many functions including:

- Defend mucosa
- Phagocytosis
- regulate of flora in intestine
- secretion of peptides with antimicrobial properties

M cells (microfold cells): Function in antigen presentation. Located above Peyer's patches.

Goblet cells: secrete mucous

Enteroendocrine cells: produce and secrete hormones including:

- secretin (S cells)
- motilin
- somatostatin (D cells)
- cholecystokinin (I cells)
- peptide YY
- glucagon-like peptide-2 (GLP-2)
- gastric inhibitory polypeptide (GIP)
- Enterochromaffin cells (APUD cells, 5-hydoxytryptamine release) carcinoid precursor

Carcinoid: tryptophan -> serotonin -> 5-HIAA (measure at urine) Tryptophan diversion may cause *pellagra* (4 D's: diarrhea, dermatitis, dementia & death)

- Serotonin is secreted by Kulchitsky cells (enterochromaffin cells) only. These cells stain + with argentafin.
- Only approximately 9% of patients ***with*** metastatic disease get Carcinoid syndrome (flushing, asthma, diarrhea, right sided heart valve lesions / dz); octreotide helps relieve symptoms
- 1/3 of pts with small bowel carcinoid have multiple primary sites
- 1/4 have metachronous adenocarcinoma
- chemo for carcinoid: streptozocin, doxorubicin, 5 FU (palliate)
- most common sites in order of frequency highest to lowest: AIR = appendix (50%), ileum, rectum
    - carcinoid involving appendix: right hemicolectomy if involves base of appendix.
      If < 2cm (and does NOT involve base), appendectomy only

Bowel rest with NGT cures 65% of partial SBO and 20% of complete SBO

Terminal ileum resection & possible sequlae: decreased bile salt absorption -> therefore less colonic H2O absorption -> causes diarrhea; results in decreased B12/intrinsic factor absorption; therefore decreased binding of oxalate -> more oxalate absorbed in colon -> more oxalate stones

Patients with Crohn's dz with numerous strictures: avoid resection (and short gut), perform stricturoplasties

Fistula: decreased healing rate in presence of FRIENDS: *F* oreign body, *R* adiation, *I* BD, *E* pithelialization, *N* eoplasm, *D* istal obstruction, *S* epsis/infection

TPN proven to increase closure rate of fistulas, but not shown to increase survival

SBO due to gallstones (from cholecysto-enteric fistula):

- SBO with air in biliary tree
- "Gallstone ileus"
- fistula usually to 2nd portion of duodenum
- Remove stone to relieve SBO but leave gallbladder and fistula to decrease mortality

Arterial supply to small bowel via the SMA. Enters on mesenteric side of the jejunum & ileum. Therefore, antimesenteric side is initial area to become ischemic when blood supply decreased / poor DO2. (eg embolus, sepsis, etc.)

Maximum absorption occurs in jejunum EXCEPT for

- bile acids (occurs mostly in ileum)
- iron (duodenum)
- folate (terminal ileum)
- bile acids (ileum)

90% of water absorbed in jejunum (NOT colon). Therefore it absorbs more water than colon. However colon's primary absorptive function is to absorb water.

Celiac axis supplies foregut and portion of duodenum, and note that SMA supplies portion of duodenum and SMA is the supply to the jejunum.

Causes of bowel obstruction WITH history of previous surgery:

- Adhesions if small bowel, BUT
- Cancer if large bowel

Causes of bowel obstruction WITHOUT history of previous surgery:

- Hernia if small bowel, BUT
- Cancer if large bowel

Characteristics of macronutrient absorption in jejunum

- Absorbs carbs
    - fructose facilitated diffusion
    - galactose and glucose active.
- proteins active transport
- fat passive

Most common tumor to metastasis to small bowel: melanoma

Blind loop syndrome

- due to bacterial overgrowth which causes B12 consumption
- Treatment is B12 and tetracyclin or augmentin

GIST (GastroIntestinal Stromal Tumor)

- Mutation in c-kit gene which produces tyrosine kinase
- mesenchymal tumor
- typically presents as GI bleed
- treatment with tyrosine kinase inhibitor Gleevec (imatinib mesylate) and resection with negative margins by frozen section

Appendicitis with suspected Crohn's

- leave active Crohn's elsewhere in bowel alone
- if appendix not involved: appendectomy so diagnosis not in doubt at future
- if appendix is involved: don't remove owing to chance of complication

Terminal ileum disease in Crohn's leads to inability to reabsorb bile into enterohepatic circulation, therefore free cholesterol turns into stones in the gallbladder of Crohn's patients.

Characteristics of Enterocytes

- primary fuel source is glutamine
- normal enterocyte lives for a little more than 2 days
- columnar and are principal cells of the villus
- found in the mucosa of the small and large bowel
- absorb a variety of nutrients including Ca, Fe and H_2O

Approximately 80% of ingested vitamin K is absorbed from the small bowel into the intestinal lymph

Arterial Blood Supply of Duodenum

- main blood supply to duodenum is from the superior and inferior pancreaticoduodenal arteries, branches of the gastroduodenal and superior mesenteric arteries, respectively

- The proximal half of the duodenum supplied by the superior pancreaticoduodenal artery and the distal half by the inferior pancreaticoduodenal artery
- These anastomose to form anterior and posterior arterial arcades between the duodenum and the pancreas
- The superior part of the duodenum may also be supplied by
  - The supraduodenal artery, arising from the common hepatic or gastroduodenal
  - The right gastric artery
  - The right gastroepiploic artery
  - The gastroduodenal artery. These vessels often anastomose with each other.

Characteristics of Migratory Motor Complex of the Small Bowel

- Seen during fasting
- Phase I has little or no contractile activity or electric spikes
- Phase II has intermittent spike activity & intermittent smooth muscle contraction
- Phase III shows maximum spike activity on every slow wave. Regular, strong contractile activity seen. (Motilin acts here.)
- Phase IV is a period of intermittent spike activity. Very brief.
- This serves as a transition phase between the phase of regular contractile activity and the quiescent phase.
- The duration of an entire cycle is approximately 90-120 minutes.
- Each phase starts in the distal esophagus, stomach, and duodenum and migrates down the small intestine. Migration takes approx 2 hours.
- Complexes are present only in the fasted state they have no apparent role in the mixing or propulsion of ingested meals.
- Function may be to clear the small bowel of residual foods, secretions, and desquamated cells during time between meals (interdigestive state).
- The MMC may also serve to limit the overgrowth of bacteria in the distal small bowel.
- Phase III of MMC includes
  - increased secretion of pepsin
  - increased secretion of hydrochloric acid by the stomach
  - increased secretion of amylase and bicarbonate by the pancreas.
- increasing duodenal output of bile acid and bilirubin during Phase II of the MMC.

Adult intussusception often has malignant leadpoint

- The intussussCIPIENS is the part of the bowel that is the reCIPIENT of another piece.
- The other part of the bowel involved is the intussussceptum

Colorectal

Development begins during the fourth gestational week

Except for the distal anal canal from ectoderm, colon is endoderm. Dentate line is dividing line between this ectoderm and endoderm

R colon and proximal transverse colon (2/3) are SMA supplied and come from midgut

Distal 1/3 transverse colon, L colon, sigmoid colon, and rectum (proximal) are IMA supplied and come from hindgut

Marginal artery of Drummond: runs along colon at margin and is a collateral between IMA and SMA

Arc of Riolan: direct, short connection between IMA and SMA

Watershed areas where hypotension may cause ischemia

- Griffith's point: at splenic flexure. SMA and IMA junction
- Sudeck's point: at rectum/rectosigmoid area. Superior rectal and middle rectal area.

Urogenital sinus divided from rectum during development. Occurs by urorectal septum formation.

While sigmoid and transverse colon are intraperitoneal, R and L colon are retroperitoneal.

Colonocytes use butyrate (fuel of the colonocyte). Main nutrient of colonocytes is short chain fatty acids.

Colon absorbs H20 (up to 5L per day) but again small bowel absorbs more H20. Does so via passive absorption.

Colon secretes K+ and reabsorbs Na+ and water.

Four histologic layers superficial to deep: serosa, muscularis propria (circular muscle layer), submucosa, mucosa (columnar epithelium).

Plicae semilunares: form haustra. These are transverse bands along colon.

Actively absorbs sodium, choride, and potassium.

Bacteria in colon produce ammonia and fatty acids.

Gross anatomic layers (superficial to deep)

- Serosa
  Stops at level of peritoneal reflection (low / mid rectum)

- Outer longitudinal muscle
  - In rectum, the longitudinal muscle is entire circumference of bowel
  - Elsewhere, longitudinal muscle comprises the tenia coli which coalesce at base of appendix and more distally splay out toward distal sigmoid.
  - Tenia coli are 3 muscle bands that run longitudinally along colon. At junction of rectum and sigmoid, these broaden and encompass circumference of bowel.
- Inner circular muscle
  Forms internal anal at level of anal canal. Internal sphincter is involuntary.

- Submucosa
- Mucosa
  Includes epithelium, lamina propria, and muscularis mucosa

External anal sphincter is voluntary, comprised of striated muscle, and contiguous with levator ani muscle.

Fascial layers near colon with unique names

- Waldeyer's fascia
  - Attaches to presacral fascia
  - Attaches to fascia propria of mesorectum anteriorly
- Denonvillier's fascia
  - In males separates rectum from seminal vesicles and prostate
  - In females separates rectum from vagina
- Presacral fascia
  Covers venous plexus in presacral area

Colon vs. small bowel

- Colon has haustra which, unlike plicae circulares, are not circumfrential.
- Colon has appendices epiploicae
- Colon has tenia coli (outer longitudinal muscle)
- Colon has intestinal glands (such as Crypts of Lieberkuhn) which are deeper than those of the small bowel.
- Colon lacks villi, small bowl has those.

Vascular supply

- SMA and IMA supply midgut and hindgut regions listed above
- Also middle hemorrhoidal artery from iliacs supplies portion of rectum
- Also inferior hemorrhoidal artery from pudendal supplies portion of rectum
- Watershed area at splenic flexure is vulnerable to ischemia
- In contrast, superior, middle, and inferior rectal arteries supply rectum making ischemia less likely
- Marginal artery of Drummond connects branches that supply colon

Internal anal sphincter is innervated by sympathetic and parasympathetics, while external anal sphincter is innervated via branch of pudendal (inferior rectal nerve). So external sphincter is under conscious control.

Rectoanal reflex occurs when feces reach rectum. Internal anal sphincter and pelvic floor relax. External anal sphincter contracts. Feces approach anus and anoderm.

Acute Appendicitis

- More common in men
- Typically seen in 2nd to 4th decades
- Affects approximately 7% of the population
- Due to occlusion of appendiceal lumen, most commonly due to lymphoid hyperplasia in adults. Other causes include fecalith and tumor.
- In older patients, incidence of tumor significantly increases (However still less common than lymphoid hyperplasia.) This is why appendicitis in older people should increase clinical suspicion of underlying appendiceal tumor.
- Elderly patients, pregnant patients, and children under 5 years of age present late with acute appendicitis owing to their atypical symptoms.
- High grade fever, symptom onset > 24 hours previously, or generalized peritonitis should increase clinical suspicion for perforation. Notice that elderly patients (who present late) are typically more commonly perforated.
- Classic history (often not seen in elderly)
  - Early on, non-specific abdominal discomfort, nausea, fever, anorexia.
  - Later, peri-umbilical pain is present and shifts to the RLQ at McBurney's point.
- Sometimes pain may be demonstrated in RLQ by palpation of LLQ. This is called Rovsing's sign. Or with hip flexion (psoas sign). Or with internally rotating the R leg (obturator sign).
- Lab tests may demonstrate a mild leukocytosis with or without left shift.
- CT scans are often used in addition to exam owing to approximately 95% sensitivity. Classic findings include:
  - Enlarged appendix with enhancement (> 6mm)
  - Fecalith
  - Wall thickening
  - Fat stranding

- Ultrasound is especially useful in children and pregnant women given radiation exposure considerations, although it is less sensitive compared to CT
- MRI is especially useful in pregnant women to assist in diagnosing appendicitis in order to minimize radiation effects.
- If phlegmon or abscess, delay resection, give antibiotics, and perform interval appendectomy.
- 15% negative appendectomy rate despite current advances in imaging and adjunct tests
- Treatment is appendectomy
  Use tenia coli to locate base of appendix. They will come together over base of appendix.

Carcinoid

- Most common malignancy of appendix
- 90% or more of cases are at appendix or distal ileum
- From enterochromaffin cells
- Usually found incidentally with appendectomy
- May be found with obstruction too or pain
- If you happen to suspect it, confirm with serum and urine serotonin (usually elevated) or chromogranin A. Octreotide scan may localize. Path shows stains positive for chromogranin A as well. However, as mentioned, usually found incidentally.
- Only about 10% of cases or less are associated with carcinoid syndrome (see earlier section on carcinoid syndrome)
- Most are < 2 cm at near appendiceal tip; however, again:
    - If base involved, needs right hemicolectomy no matter what size.
    - If > 2 cm, needs right hemicolectomy
    - If there are mets to liver, no matter what size and whether involves base, needs R hemicolectomy
- Resect hepatic mets (debulk) if present
- Octreotide is used to treat symptoms if mets
- Streptozocin, doxorubicin are used as chemotherapy for palliation if unresectable mets.

Typhlitis

- May masquerade as appendicitis
- Neutropenic enterocolitis that affects the terminal ileum, cecum, & right colon.
- When patient has leukemia or is immunosuppressed (eg AIDS, chemo, transplant) consider this diagnosis
- Presents as diahrrea, fever, emesis, RLQ pain, etc.
- Useful to calculate absolute neutrophil count (ANC)
- Treatment is medical and includes NGT, NPO, IV fluid, and antibiotics. May treat ANC with neupogen as well.

Large bowel obstruction

- Whether patient has had previous surgery or has NOT had previous surgery: most common cause of large bowel obstruction is cancer
- Trostle's rule: don't let a patient with any question of large bowel obstruction leave the hospital without an operation unless it's due to Ogilvie's. Don't see them in the ER and discharge them with a partial colon obstruction, etc.
- 15% of intestinal obstruction cases
- other causes include diverticulitis, volvulus, impaction, post op adhesions, hernia, pseudo-obstruction.
- Emesis is more commonly a later finding owing to presence of ileocecal valve
- Lab tests are often non-specific
- Dilated colon without rectal air suggests mechanical obstruction while presence of air suggests pseudo-obstruction
- CT imaging very useful to make diagnosis.
- Fluid resuscitate, place NGT, correct electrolytes
- Unlike small bowel obstruction where NGT and wait is often first-line treatment, surgical intervention is first line treatment for large bowel obstruction.
- Unless it's due to Ogilvie's (pseudo-obstruction) large bowel obstruction requires operation. (Not necessarily emergent but generally on same hospital stay. See Trostle's rule.)
- For pseudo-obstruction (Ogilvie's syndrome), decompression and neostigmine may be utilized.
- Mortality rate for patients with large bowel obstruction is approximately 20%

Volvulus

- Cause of about 5% of large bowel obstructions
- Closed loop which is obstruction due to twist of bowel more than 180 degrees on its mesentery. Results in obstruction at two locations that are included where bowel twists.
- Risk factors include being bedridden, chronic constipation, megacolon, pregnancy, redundant segment.
- Typically seen in patients > 70 years old.
- Cecal bascule is folding of cecum anteromedially on itself.
- Cecal volvulus occurs when cecum rotates around ileocolic vessels and is owing to twisting of mesentery.
- Volvulus may and often does result in ischemia. Abdominal pain and hemodynamic instability may be seen.
- Classic sign of sigmoid volvulus on xray is "bent inner tube" narrowing into "bird's beak".
- "Coffee bean" appearance may be seen on xray in patients with cecal volvulus.
- If nonstrangulated sigmoid volvulus, may perform endoscopic decompression with placement of rectal tube. Surgery is typically indicated even with successful reduction to avoid recurrence. Urgent surgical intervention should be performed for sigmoid volvulus if there is a question of strangulation.
- Cecal volvulus requires emergent surgery which may include cecopexy or right hemicolectomy. Cecostomy is an option but carries a high risk of recurrence and so is performed in select patients only.

Diverticulae

- Most common disease of the colon
- Greater than 90% of the time affects the sigmoid colon of geriatric patients
- Obesity, low fiber diet, tobacco use, constipation, and sedentary lifestyle are all risk factures
- Herniation of mucosa at weak areas in muscularis externa. Areas where blood vessels enter and leave are some of these weak areas.
- Diverticulosis is presence of these non-inflamed lesions
- Diverticulitis is when inflammation is present at these diverticuli, often due to a microperforation. Complications include frank perforation, stricture (long term), obstruction, or gross perforation.
- Diverticulosis may bleed and present as bright red blood per rectum
- Remember: "-osis bleeds, -itis perfs".
- Diverticulitis typically causes lower quadrant pain with associated leukocytosis and fever.
- WBC is non-specific. CT scan is useful to demonstrate whether diverticulitis, diverticulosis, and / or a related complication is present.
- Diverticulosis
    - High fiber diet
    - Bleeds usually resolve spontaneously but requires surgery if persists or recurs
- Diverticulitis
    - Typically treated with bowel rest and oral antibiotics
    - Drain if abscess present
    - Operate emergently if perforation and significant free air. Hartmann's procedure is resection of diseased portion of colon, abdominal lavage, and end colostomy. Note that proximal extent of colonic resection is to the level of induration and NOT all of the colon that demonstrates diverticulae.
    - Perforation with abscess often amenable to percutaneous drainage.
    - If there is an episode of complicated diverticulitis, eg abscess, elective resection at a later date is indicated. Other indications to operate include young patient (because will likely have many more episodes and issues throughout life), immunosuppressed patients, or after multiple (typically two) attacks.

Lower GI bleed

- When you see blood per rectum, remember that UPPER GI bleed is most common cause
- Lower GI bleed (LGIB) more common in men
- Average age at diagnosis is 60s to late 70s
- Lower GI bleeding is defined as bleeding distal to the ligament of Treitz (LOT)
- Angiodyplasia, diverticulosis, Meckel's, ischemia, inflammatory bowel disease, infection (eg E. Coli or C. Diff), cancer, or hemorrhoids are all potential causes.
- Lower GI bleed usually stops spontaneously
- Transfusion of more than 6U PRBCs within first 24 hours of stay predicts need for operative intervention
- Remember, an NGT is one of the first steps to localize a GI bleed to UGI or LGI bleed.
- An NGT negative for UGI is one that demonstrates no blood but DOES demonstrate bile. Just because an NGT does NOT demonstrate blood does NOT mean an UGI bleed is ruled out.
- And even when an NGT is truly negative (shows bile and NO blood) it is NOT a perfect test to rule out UGI bleeding.
- If NGT is positive for UGI bleed, perform EGD, establish source, and treat as appropriate.
- If NGT does not demonstrate UGI bleed, perform colonoscopy.
    - If source visualized, injection / thermal therapy.
    - If GI source not visualized, and if "fast bleed" (more than 1 mL / min), perform angiography with angioembolization if possible. (Localizes and treats.)
    - If GI source not visualized, and if not a "fast bleed" perform tagged red blood cell scan to localize.
    - If severe bleeding present, and this prevents visualization during colonoscopy...
        - if "fast bleed" (more than 1 mL / min), perform angiography with angioembolization if possible. (Localizes and treats.)
        - If not a "fast bleed" performed tagged red blood cell scan to localize.
        - Yes, this is similar to nonvisualization portion above.
- If bleeding is uncontrolled after angioembolization attempted, patient requires surgical intervention.
- If bleeding is controlled, but no colonic source is identified, evaluate small bowel with capsule endoscopy or other technique.

Inflammatory bowel disease

- Crohn's and Ulcerative Colitis (UC)
- Underlying causes for each are not clear
- Extra-intestinal manifestations of both
  - Primary sclerosing cholangitis (more especially with UC)
  - Erythema nodosum
  - Pyoderma gangrenosum
  - Sacro-ileitis
  - Arthritis
  - Uveitis & scleritis
  - Pericarditis
  - Ankylosing spondylitis
- Patients with inflammatory bowel disease require annual colonscopies starting after disease has been present for 8-10 years owing to risk of colorectal cancer.
- Specifics of ulcerative colitis (UC)
  - Typically affects patients in 3rd or 7th decade
  - 10 / 100,000 is incidence
  - Ashkenazi Jewish descent is risk factor
  - Interestingly, tobacco DECREASES risk
  - Diarrhea, blood per rectum, abdominal pain, fever are typical symptoms
  - Colonoscopy with biopsy makes diagnosis
  - Depth of involvement includes mucosa and submucosa
  - Involvement of bowel wall is transmural
  - Path features friable mucosa, crypt abscesses, pseudopolyps, and continuous involvement of bowel (NO skip lesions)
  - Bleeding, toxic megacolon, fulminant UC, colorectal cancer and extra-intestinal manifestations may be seen
  - Extra-intestinal manifestations include aphthous ulcer, iritis, uveitis, episcleritis, seronegative arthritis, ankylosing spondylitis, sacroilitis, erythema nodosum, pyoderma gangrenosum, DVT & PE, autoimmune hemolytic anemia, clubbing, primary sclerosing cholangitis
- Some extra-intestinal manifestations seen with UC get better with colectomy eg anemia, arthritis, ocular issues.
- Some manifestations of UC do NOT get better with colectomy: primary sclerosing cholangitis, ankylosing spondylitis
- Half of pyoderma gangrenosum patients get better with colectomy.

- Treatment for an acute attack of UC may include steroids, 5-ASA, Infliximab (severe disease), cyclosporine (for steroid refractory disease)
- Maintenance treatment for UC may include sulfasalazine or 5-ASA. May include 6-mercaptopurine / azathioprine
- Subtotal colectomy / proctocolectomy with end ileostomy is performed if emergency surgery is required in UC
- Total proctocolectomy with ileal pouch and anal anastomosis is most common procedure in UC if patient is candidate for elective procedure. However, total proctocolectomy and permanenet ileostomy may also be performed in this context.
- Specifics of Crohn's disease
    - 2nd and 6th decade is peak incidence
    - affects around 3/100,000 people
    - Ashkenazi Jewish descent is risk factor
    - Tobacco increases risk
    - Unlike UC that is seen in the colon, Crohn's is more commonly seen anywhere along the GI tract. Most common in the terminal ileum.
    - Obstruction, abdominal pain, weight loss, diarrhea, bleeding, and fever may be seen
    - Colonscopy and biopsy may give diagnosis. If present in small bowel (and not colon) CT scan with oral contrast may be useful
    - Involvement of bowel wall is transmural
    - Skip lesions seen. Non-caseating granulomas, fistulae (sometimes perianal), cobblestoning, and strictures are seen
    - Toxic megacolon, small bowel cancers, colorectal cancer, and extra-intestinal manifestations, are all seen
    - Perianal disease is treated with flagyl.
    - Treatment for maintenance and acute attacks is similar to ulcerative colitis.
    - Elective surgical intervention involves resection of diseased portions of bowel.
    - Stricturoplasty is used when possible to minimize the risk of short bowel syndrome.

Carcinoid of the colon and rectum

- Approximately 15% of carcinoid tumors
- Low rectal carcinoids
    - Greater than 2 cm: wide excision with negative margins
    - Less than 2 cm or any size with invasion of muscularis propria: perform APR
- Colonic or high rectal carcinoids
    - Greater than 1 cm: resection
    - Less than 1 cm: polypectomy may be performed

Colorectal syndromes associated with hamartomatous polyps

- Peutz-Jegher:
  - Autosomal dominant
  - polyps are hamartomatous
  - Polyps typically in ileum or jejunum. May also be in rectum.
  - Buccal mucosa is hyperpigmented
  - Increased risk of adenomatous degeneration and increase risk of extra-intestinal cancers
  - Breast, testis/ovary, pancreas, biliary
- Cowden's syndrome
  - PTEN mutation
  - Autosomal dominant
  - GI polyps
  - Leiomyomas of uterus
  - Breast and thyroid cancers
  - Mucocutaneous lesions
- Juvenile polyposis
  - Autosomal dominant
  - Polyps throughout GI tract
  - Colorectal cancer risk is increased
- Cronkite-Canada syndrome
  - Sporadic
  - Dystrophic nails
  - Hyperpigmentation
  - Alopecia

Colorectal cancer

- Equal incidence in men and women
- Second leading cause of cancer death in US
- Age > 50 is risk factor
- History of colonic adenoma is a risk factor
- Inflammatory bowel disease is a risk factor
- Family history of colon cancer is a risk factor
- APC, DCC, p53 and k-ras are main gene mutations
- Adenomas are premalignant. Tubular adenomas are most common, villous adenomas have increased risk of cancer compared to tubulovillous and tubular.
- Change in stool caliber, rectal bleeding, and obstruction are some of many signs
- Increased carcinoembryonic antigen (CEA) is sometimes seen
- Digital rectal exam (DRE) and fecal occult blood testing (FOBT) are useful
- CT colonoscopy, colonoscopy, and barium enema are useful to make diagnosis.
- Tools for staging include endoscopic ultrasound (EUS), MRI pelvis, and CT.
- Resections for colon cancer should include at least 12 lymph nodes to allow for correct staging
- Treatment for rectal cancer is DIFFERENT than colon cancer and includes radiation and chemotherapy. Colon cancer receives chemo ONLY.
- Need colonoscopy as part of staging to be sure there's no synchronous lesion.

- T portion of TNM staging is based on invasiveness not tumor size:
    - Tis = lesion does NOT invade submucosa
    - T1 = invades submucosa
    - T2 = invades muscularis propria
    - T3 = invades into subserosa / non-peritonealized pericolic or perirectal tissue
    - T4 = invades adjacent organ
    - N portion of TNM staging is generally related to the number of nodes involved
    - N0 = no nodes involved
    - N1 = 1-3 nodes involved
    - N2 = 4 or more nodes involved
    - N3 = lymph node adjacent to major vessel is positive
    - M portion
    - M0 metastatic disease absent
    - M1 positive mets
- Best for T and N status is TRUS (trans-retal ultrasound) if lesion is accessible
- Stage 1 is TisN0M0
- Stage 2 is T1 or T2 N0M0
- Stage 3 is any tumor with positive nodes but no metastasis
- Stage 4 is any tumor with or without nodes but positive metastasis
    - Most common site for mets is liver. If resectable and isolated 5 year survival is 35%
    - Lung mets (isolated and resectable) with 25% 5 year survival rate
    - Isolated liver or lung mets should receive resection
    - Rectal cancer may metastasize to spine directly via Batson's plexus

- Alternative staging for colon cancer is Duke's classification
    - Stage A: submucosal invasion
    - Stage B: invasion into muscularis propria with negative nodes
    - Stage C: positive nodes
    - Stage D: presence of metastasis or invasion into adjacent structures
- Less commonly used that TNM classification
- Each TNM stage aligns with a Duke's classification
- Five year survival by stage:
    - Stage 1(Duke's A) = 95%
    - Stage 2 (Duke's B) = 85%
    - Stage 3 (Duke's C) = 30-60%
    - Stage 4 (Duke's D) = 5%

Amsterdam criteria are used to determine whether patient has hereditary non-polyposis colon cancer (HNPCC)

- Also known as 3, 2, 1 rule
- Confirmation that tumor is NOT familial adenomatous polyposis (FAP) related by biopsy / testing
- 3 or more relatives, including at least one first degree relative, with a known HNPCC
- 2 or more generations affected in family
- 1 or more affected patient who is less than 50 years old

Colon cancer syndromes

- 20% of patients with colon cancer have a family history of colon cancer
- HNPCC (Lynch Syndrome)
  - Due to mutations in DNA mismatch repair genes, eg hMLH1, hMSH2
  - Lifetime risk of colon cancer is 85%
  - Lynch 1 leads to onset of colorectal cancer at a young age
  - Lynch 2 give increased risk of GI malignancy such as stomach, small bowel, pancreas, biliary, endometrial, and genitourinary tumors
  - Annual colonoscopy starting at 20-25 years or 10 years earlier than age at which youngest family member diagnosed with colorectal cancer. For females with Lynch syndrome, screening recommendations include transvaginal ultrasound annually at 25-35 years or annual endometrial biopsy.
- Turcot's syndrome
  - Due APC gene mutation (on chromosome 5q)
  - Increased risk of colorectal cancer and brain tumors. Colonic adenomas seen.
  - Screening recommendations are same as for familial adenomatous polyposis (FAP) as beneath.
- Gardner's syndrome
  - Due to APC gene mutation on chromosome 5q as with Turcot's
  - Increased risk of colorectal cancer with desmoid tumors, osteoid tumors, and skin cysts. Colonic adenomas seen.
  - Screening as with FAP as beneath.

- FAP
    - APC mutation (chromosome 5q)
    - Colon ademonas seen and lifetime risk of colorectal cancer is 100%.
    - Increased risk of multiple other tumors as well including periampullary tumors, thyroid tumors, and adrenocortical tumors.
    - Flexible sigmoidoscopy annually at 10 -15 years old.
    - Upper endoscopy each 1-3 years after age 25
    - Diagnosis of FAP requires surgery
    - Procedure chosen depends on whether rectum is involved, whether cancer is already present, and also patient age
    - Outcomes for resection in FAP patients are similar to colorectal cancer cases that are NOT related to a hereditary syndrome if resection is prophylactic in nature when performed.
    - If cancer present, subtotal colectomy or segmental colectomy is performed. And total abdominal hysterectomy with bilateral salpingo-oopherectomy is often added in women with Lynch 2 owing to risk of eventual cancer in reproductive organs.
    - Otherwise, total proctocoletomy with ileostomy, total abdominal colectomy with ileorectal anastomosis, or total proctocolectomy with J pouch (aka Ileal Pouch Anal Anastamosis [IPAA] is chosen.

Most common causes of acute pain at anus are external hemorrhoid thrombosis, perianal abscess, and anal fissure.

Condyloma acuminata

- Due to human papilloma virus (HPV)
- Fulgaration is treatment (lazer or alternative)

Anal fissure

- Ulcer or tear which is distal to dentate line in the anoderm
- Typically posterior and in midline
- May be related to insufficient fiber in diet
- Pain and bleeding with defecation
- Caused by hypertonic internal anal sphincter
- At times, may see sentinel pile distal to the ulcer / tear in anoderm
- May see hypertrophy of anal papillae proximally
- Exam makes diagnosis, and internal anal sphincter spasm is also seen
- Should perform endoscopy / anoscopy to rule out more serious underlying condition
- Treatment includes stool softeners, nifedipine ointment, Sitz baths. When medical treatment fails, requires lateral internal anal sphincterotomy or injection of botox into sphincter
- Note that lateral internal sphincterotomy may give incontinence

Hemorrhoids

- Risk factors include things that increase intra-abdominal pressure, eg: obesity, pregnancy, needing to strain with defecation
- Common positions are left lateral, right anterolateral, and right posterolateral
- Due to engorged anal submucosa cushions and NOT varicose veins
- Types include internal and external
- Internal are Insensate. Also are superior to dentate line. (Therefore columnar or transitional epithelium.) Staged by degree of prolapse.
    - First degree: no prolapse
    - Second degree: spontaneously reducing prolapse
    - Third degree: prolapse that requires reduction
    - Fourth degree: prolapse that can not be reduced
- External hemorrhoids are beneath the dentate line (therefore squamous epithelial tissue) in the innervated anoderm. These hurt.
- May present as red blood per rectum. May cause bothersome swelling and difficulties with hygiene in area.
- Digital rectal exam, anoscopy, and sigmoidoscopy help make diagnosis.
- Screen for colon cancer with endoscopy if patient is less than 40 years old, unusual symptoms are noted, or there is a family history of colon CA.
- Treatments include Sitz baths, stool softeners, increasing water and fiber intake, creams, ointments.
- Many options for treatment exist if medical management fails, including rubber band ligation, sclerotherapy, and hemorrhoidectomy.
- If large hemorrhoids and/or significant external component, perform surgical hemorrhoidectomy.
- Office excision may be performed for isolated, thrombosed external hemorrhoid that presents less than 4-5 days from onset. Fiber and Sitz baths may be used for patients with later presentation.

Pilonidal cyst

- Infected hair containing sinus. Usually seen in gluteal cleft but may also be seen on hands of hairstylists.
- Usually seen in men
- Diagnosed on exam.
- Treated with incision and resection of cyst lining with marsupialization or closure

Proctitis

- HPV, CMV, UC, Crohn's, radiation, C diff, STDs...all can cause inflammation of the anorectum.
- Treatment is based on the underlying cause.

Anal fistula

- Occurs between anal canal and peri-anal skin
- Inter, trans, supra, or extra-sphincteric are classifications.
- Starts as abscess in a crypt gland of dentate line which becomes an interphincteric abscess and then peri-anal abscess
- Although most are idiopathic, Crohn's may be a cause
- Most are anterior or posterior
- Lateral fistula are more often due to less common causes such as HIV or TB
- Presents as drainage from an external opening, often in a location where there was a perianal abscess that "never healed".
- Goodsall's rule (sometimes called the "dog rule"): more anterior openings tract directly into anal canal, and posterior openings take a curved tract into the anal canal. Dogs' noses are straight and their tails are curved, so Goodsall's rule is sometimes nicknamed the dog rule.
- Treatment is fistulotomy, and remember that incontinence is a potential complication if sphincter is divided. So fistulae that may involve external sphincter often receive a staged fistulotomy with a non-cutting seton.
- Remember that Crohn's and malignancy may cause fistulae. These should be considered before treating anorectal complaints.

Rectal prolapse

- Usually seen in women > 60 years old
- Rectal wall protrudes through anus and presents as incontinence, vaginal / uterine prolapse, cystocele, enterocele, or constipation.
- Often associated with weak pelvic floor
- True prolapse (full thickness) demonstrates circumferential mucosal folds
- False prolapse (mucosa only) demonstrates radial folds
- The rectum may become ischemic which causes tenderness. This is rare.
- Colonscopy or contrast enema should be performed to rule out underlying lesion
- For good operative candidates, laparotomy and rectopexy (with or without sigmoid resection) is performed
- For others, rectosigmoidectomy via perineal approach (Altemeier procedure) is performed or Delorme's procedure (perineal approach with resection of mucosa and submucosa of prolapsed segment only)

Anal cancer

- Usually squamous cell cancer from HPV infection
- Adenocarcinoma is 10% of cases only and prognosis is worse
- Most common in young male patients who engage in receptive anal intercourse
- HIV, Crohn's, Hodgkin's, HSV2, and STDs are other risk factors.
- May be asymptomatic or demonstrate pain, puritis, rectal bleeding, or anal fullness.
- Exam may reveal anal mass with or without lymphadenopathy
- Colonscopy with biopsy reveals diagnosis. Staging performed with CT abdomen and pelvis.
- Nigro protocol (5FU and mitomycin with radiation) is used for larger lesions or anal canal lesions. Small lesions or those on perianal skin receive wide local excision.
- Abdomino-perineal resection (APR) is used for recurrent or persistent disease after these treatments.
- 5 year survival is 60-70%
- rarely basal cell CA
  treatment is wide local excision. Only 3mm margin needed. APR rarely necessary...typically only if sphincter is involved.

Miscellaneous facts from colorectal...

External anal sphincter is puborectalis muscle and is under conscious control. Internal pudendal nerve is innervation (inferior rectal branch). This sphincter is actually a continuation of levator ani muscle which is striated.

Internal anal sphincter is innervated by pelvic splanchnic nerves and its normal state is to be contracted. It is a continuation of muscularis propria from colon.

Colonic inertia is significant slow transit time. Patients may need subtotal colectomy.

Stump pouchitis (aka diversion or disuse pouchitis) is treated with short chain fatty acid enemas

Infectious pouchitis is treated with flagyl

False positive guiac (fecal occult blood screen) with cimetidine, beef, vitamin C, or iron.

Polypectomy performed by colonoscopy and pathology shows T1 cancer

- If 2mm clear margin, poly is well differentiated, there is no vascular / lymph invasion...nothing else to do. Continue surveillance
- If ANY of those criteria are violated, needs colon resection

Overall screening recommendations for colorectal cancer: colonscopy starting at 50YOA for normal risk patients, 40 YOA (or ten years before youngest case) if family history colon cancer. Exceptions as noted in hereditary colon cancer syndromes as above.

Low rectal villous adenoma with atypia: transanal resection of as much as possible. APR only if cancer is present.

- Pathology shows T1 lesion after transanal for villous polyp: no need for further resection if 2mm margins are clear AND no vascular / lymph invasion. If there is either or both of those findings, APR / LAR.
- Pathology shows T2 lesion after transanal for villous polyp: APR or LAR.

Medications & Anesthesia

Methoxyfluorane has renal toxicity.

Halothane

- may cause cardiac arrhythmias.
- hepatotoxic

Succinylcholine is the only depolarizing agent used; generalized contractions, hyperkalemia in burn patients, fast on/off; risk of aspiration, glaucoma

Ketamine increases cardiac work, O2 use, secretions, BP. No respiratory depression. Does give hallucinations

Clindamycin prolongs neuromuscular blockade

Demerol should be avoided in patients on MAOIs

Octreotide: long-acting somatostatin analog

Omeprazole: blocks Na/H ATPase; associated with enterochromaffin hyperplasia in rats. No evidence of carcinogenesis in humans. Increases risk for Cdif and pneumonia in certain patients.

Digoxin: glycoside, inhibits Na-K ATPase and increases calcium in heart. Slows AV conduction. Inotrope but does not increase O2 consumption. Associated with ischemic gut because of decreased splanchnic flow.

Amrinone: is a phosphodiesterase inhibitor. Also and inotrope, increases CO, decreases SVR

Metyrapone and Aminoglutethimide: give a "medical adrenalectomy"

Leuprolide: gives a "medical orchiectomy"

Vasopressin: reduces splanchnic blood blow, portal flow by around 40%. Useful in GIB, give with ß-blocker to avoid angina.

Sodium nitroprusside relaxes arteries and veins. May cause cyanide toxicity

Nitroglycerin primarily relaxes veins

Aspirin irreversibly binds *cyclooxygenase*, effective for life of platelets (which is around 7 days)

Indomethacin blocks prostaglandin production, used to close PDA (effective approximately 70%). Decreases renal blood flow

Misoprostil may be used to replace PGE2 for patient on NSAIDS to reduce peptic ulcer disease

First Order Kinetics in Drug Dosage

In first order kinetics a constant fraction of the drug is eliminated per unit time. The rate of elimination is proportional to the amount of drug in the body. So the half life is equal to the rate of elimination.

Calculation of drug loading dose: Volume of Distribution X Desired Steady State Plasma Concentration.

Volume of Distribution: Dose / plasma concentration.

Malignant Hyperthermia

- May be caused by succinylcholine, inhaled anesthesia, amide local anesthetics (bupivicaine and lidocaine). Due to genetic mutation in the sarcoplasmic reticulum.
- Often seen: fever, tachycardia, rigidity, skin mottling, cyanosis. Metabolic acidosis and hyperkalemia.
- Stop anesthesia and give dantrolene. Associated hyperkalemia and acidosis may be treated with insulin and bicarbonate.

Succinylcholine issues

- non-competitive depolarizing agent (only depolarizing agent used) binds to acetyl choline receptor on muscle. First activates then paralyzes because of binding to receptor.
- contraindicated in renal disease because elevates K+ level. Burns, Rhabdo, Spinal Cord Injury, pseudocholinesterase deficiency, musculoskeletal disorders (myasthenia gravis etc) also contraindicated.
- Makes glaucoma worse. Works on striated muscle. Bradycardia, arrhythmias and malignant hyperthermia.
- The major complication of succinylcholine is arrhythmia from a high release of K+ stores causing arrhythmias and asystole.

Propofol: amnesia, sedation, some analgesia, may cause hypotension.

Atracurium

- nondepolarizing agent (again sux is only depolarizing agent used) that undergoes Hoffman Elimination and so is used in kidney / liver disease.
- causes histamine release.

Etomidate may cause adrenal insufficiency.

Pancuronium causes tachycardia.

Vecuronium causes NO histamine release and does NOT cause autonomic effects

Toradol causes Bleeding, Renal Failure, Ulcers.

Ketamine

- Do not use in cardiac ischemia or increased intracranial pressure.
- causes hallucinations and depresses cardiac function
- use in hypotensive patient or in respiratory disease because it is a smooth muscle reactant.

First pass metabolism involves metabolism by the liver. Sublingual and rectal route have higher bioavailability than drugs taken orally.

For drug absorption into CSF: must be a lipid soluble, non-ionized drug.

Coumadin, penicillin, and *many* other drugs bind to albumin.

Zero order kinetics: elimination does not depend on dose of drug. A set amount is eliminated over each time interval no matter what dose given.

First order kinetics: amount eliminated is related to the amount of drug given

Drug steady state and ½ lives: 5 half lives required to reach steady state

Volume of distribution = (amount of drug in body) / (amount of drug in blood)

Bioavailability is percentage of drug that enters circulation without being metabolized (100% for IV administration route)

Level of drug at which effect occurs in 50% of patients is called "effective dose for 50%" or ED50

Level of drug at which death occurs in 50% of patients is called "lethal dose for 50%" or LD50.

Gadolinium: do NOT use with renal insufficiency or failure because may cause nephrogenic systemic fibrosis.

Specific characteristics of metoclopramide (aka Reglan)

- Used in large doses in the treatment of nausea induced by chemotherapy
- Antidopaminergic & increases gastrointestinal motility
- Reverses nausea and vomiting caused by narcotics (i.e. postoperative vomiting)
- it may be useful before emergency surgery to promote gastric emptying
- Helps prevent aspiration by tightening lower esophageal sphincter to prevent aspiration during emergency induction of anesthesia
- Does NOT prevent motion-sickness (unlike scopolamine)
- Useful in gastroparesis in diabetic patients
- Improves response to ergotamine in treatment of migraine headaches
- Adverse reactions
    - sedation and diarrhea
    - Extrapyramidal reactions, like parkinsonian symptoms and tardive dyskinesia, have been seen when used for months or years
    - Extrapyramidal reactions reversible with diphenhydramine (Benadryl)
    - Dystonic reactions, such as oculogyric crises, trismus, torticollis, opisthotonos and akathisia are more likely in the first 72 hours of treatment.
    - More common in children, young adults, renal impairment, and with larger doses such as those seen in chemotherapy patients.
    - May increase sedative actions of CNS depressants.
    - May increase severity and frequency of extrapyramidal reactions produced by other medications, particularly phenothlazines.

- Contraindications:
    - GI obstruction, hemorrhage, or perforation.
    - Convulsive disorders
    - Pheochromocytoma
- Drug kinetics
    - renal excretion with some hepatic conjugation
    - 1/2-life with normal renal function: 4-6 hours, & not dose dependent

Cyclosporine use & complications

- Is a cyclic peptide produced by a fungus
- suppresses T-cells
- Inhibits activation of resting T-lymphocytes, resulting in inhibition of IL-2 production.
- Once the T-lymphocytes have been activated, cyclosporine is NOT effective in suppressing the immune response.
- Cyclosporine is absorbed from the GI tract. Absorption is slow and incomplete.
- Excretion is mostly through bile.
- There is an enterohepatic cycle.
- Adverse effects of cyclosporine include hirsutism, neurotoxicities, hyperkalemia, nephrotoxicity and hepatotoxicity.
- The most frequent toxic effects are nephrotoxicity, hypertension and tremors.

Lidocaine toxicity

- Lidocaine overdose produces death from either ventricular fibrillation or cardiac arrest.
- Max dose: 4-5mg/kg, 7mg/kg if given with epinephrine.
- Amides (such as bupivicaine and lidocaine) are less allergenic than the esters (such as cocaine) and may be used in patients with ester drug allergies. Esters are broken down into PABA which is highly allergenic in people.
- Perioral numbness / tingling, tinnitus these progress to CNS symptoms such as seizures followed by Vfib / cardiac arrest
- At higher levels of toxicity individuals will experience decreased hearing, disorientation, muscle twitching, convulsions, or respiratory arrest.
- Less severe side effects include sleepiness, dizziness, paresthesias, altered mental status, coma, seizures.

Quinolones

- Bactericidal
- Mechanism of action is interference with the enzyme DNA gyrase, needed for bacterial DNA replication.
- Increases theophylline levels.
- Gives increased anticoagulant effect, thought to be secondary to an alteration of hepatic metabolism.

Characteristics of high-dose fentanyl analgesia

- highly soluble lipid and approximately 100 times more potent than morphine.
- Narcotic drugs act via several receptors (mu, kappa, delta, sigma) although all of their effects cannot be explained by this mechanism alone.
- Cause pupillary constriction by inhibiting the Edinger - Westphal nucleus in the brain
- cause respiratory depression by altering brain stem response to CO2 and/or causing sedation
- cause nausea/vomiting by stimulating the chemoreceptor trigger zone in the medulla and cause decreased GI motility.
- Cardiovascular effects of narcotics include
    - moderate peripheral vasodilation and histamine release, which may cause hypotension
    - decrease heart rate by inhibition of central vagal nucleus in the medulla.
- Fentanyl in large doses is typically better tolerated than other narcotics because it causes little histamine release and also direct cardiodepressive effects are minimal.
- At high doses, opioids may cause skeletal muscle rigidity. This may make ventilation difficult without muscle relaxants.
- With fentanyl this is probably due to its rapid uptake by skeletal muscle.

Chemotherapy causing hemorrhagic cystitis

- Cyclophosphamide is associated with hemorrhagic cystitis. May occur in up to 10% of patients due to active metabolites (eg acrolein)
- The risk is decreased with 3-4 liters of fluid per day and administration of N-acetylcysteine

Peak and trough management: if peak is high lower the dose, if trough is high increase the interval

Clopidogrel: stop 5 days before surgery. Irreversibly modifies ADP receptor on platelet. Platelets live 5-7 days.

Milrinone is utilized post Coronary Artery Bypass to improve LV function in those patients who have an increased pulmonary artery pressure. Tachycardia is NOT a side effect.

Breast

Embryology

- Mammary ridges form at 4-6 weeks along ventral side of embryo from ectoderm.
- These regress in few days except for a remnant at 4th intercostal space.
- Incomplete regression may lead to polythelia (accessory nipples) or polymastia (accessory mammary glands)

Macroscopic Anatomy

- Intercostobrachial nerve (from 2nd intercostal nerve) gives sensation to medial arm. May be sacrificed in dissection.
- Long thoracic nerve: goes to serratus anterior. Injury gives winged scapula.
- Thoracodorsal nerve: goes to latissimus dorsi. Injury gives inability to do pullups and weak arm Abduction
- Medial pectoral nerve: goes to pec minor and pec major.
- Lateral pectoral nerve: goes to pec minor ONLY
- Batson's plexus are Valveless Vertebral Veins (VVV). Thought to allow direct mets from breast CA to spine.
- Blood supply: arterial supply includes the internal thoracic, axillary, and third to fifth inter- costal arteries. Venous system parallels the arterial supply (eg, internal thoracic, axillary, and third to fifth intercostal veins)

Poland syndrome: hypoplastic pectoral muscles, hypoplastic shoulder, no breast (amastia), all on same side typically right side. Patients may not know they have this until puberty. Also associated with hand abnormalities.

Mastodynia: "breast pain" may be treated with multiple different agents including: supportive bra, oral contraceptives, danazol, evening primrose oil, tamoxifen,

Mondor's disease: thrombophlebitis of superficial breast veins. Feels like cord like mass.

Breast cancer tumor sizes for TNM staging

- T1 < 2cm
- T2 2-5cm
- T3 > 5cm
- T4 skin or chest wall involvement
- 'grave signs' = peau d'orange, inflammation

Nodes staging for breast cancer TNM

- N1 + axillary nodes
- N2 matted or fixed nodes
- N3 internal mammary nodes
- NB: lymph node LEVELS are defined relative to pec minor muscle
  - Level 1: Lateral to pec minor ("level one lateral")
  - Level 2: Deep to pec minor
  - Level 3: medial to pec minor

Stage I T1; II up to T2N1 or T3N0; III T4 or N2; IV Mets (includes supraclavicular node, unlike lung CA)

Breast mets: to bone, lung, brain. (In order of decreasing frequency.)

Her 2 neu: a marker for breast CA, implies worse prognosis. *Herceptin* now available for Rx.

Erb B 2, p53, cathepsin all indicate worse prognosis

1cm tumor is approximately 5 yrs old

Tamoxifen reduces risk 50% in high risk patients but increases endometrial cancer and DVT risk

Atypical hyperplasia raises risk 4 times (only finding in fibrocystic that increases risk)

ER+PR+ is better for prognosis than ER-PR+ which is better than ER+PR- which is better than ER-PR-

DCIS 50% develop invasive carcinoma, is a *precursor*. Usually lumpectomy + RT, but mastectomy for high grade/large tumor/poor margins. 50% of DCIS recurrence is invasive marker of risk

LCIS 30-40% develop invasive carcinoma (either breast), is a , Treatment options: nothing, tamoxifen, or bilateral mastectomy

Comedo Breast CA: likely multicentric, do mastectomy. Poor prognosis

Cystosarcoma Phyllodes or 'Phyllodes tumor' only 10% malignant; Large; Rare nodal mets; As with other sarcomas, spread is *hematogenous*, not lymphatic. Rx is wide local excision, rarely mastectomy, *no* axillary node dissection

Microscopic Anatomy

- Each glandular lobe consists of tubuloalveolar epithelium arranged in lobules.
- Milk is made in the branching alveoli of the breast lobules during lactation.
- Multiple alveoli drain into a single alveolar duct, which merges with others to form 15–20 lactiferous ducts.
- Each lactiferous duct drains a breast lobe.

Indications for genetic screening for breast cancer:

- member of family with known BRCA mutation
- male relative (first, second, or third degree) with breast cancer
- Personal history of breast cancer.
- Personal history of ovarian cancer.
- Diagnosis of breast cancer ≤ 40 years of age (+/- family history of disease)
- Personal history of male breast cancer especially in the setting of ≥ 1 of the following criteria:
  - male relative (first, second, or third degree) with breast cancer
  - female relative (first, second, or third degree) with breast or ovarian cancer
- Diagnosis of breast cancer ≤ 50 years of age OR
  two 1° breast cancers (bilateral disease or ipsilateral 1° tumors) and ≤ 1 first, second, or third degree relative with breast cancer ≤ 50 years and/or first, second, or third degree relative with ovarian cancer, or personal history of ovarian cancer

Obesity and cirrhosis are associated with hyperestrogenemia, resulting in stimulation of breast tissue.

BRCA 1

- chromosome 17q
- autosomal dominant inheritance
- Increased risk of breast cancer (80%)
- Increased risk of ovarian (40%) cancer
- early disease onset and bilateral
- Prophylactic mastectomies & bilateral salpingo-oophorectomy considered.

BRCA 2

- chromosome 13q
- normally involved in DNA repair
- Increased risk of breast cancer (60%), including male breast cancer
- Increased risk of ovarian cancer (15–25%)

Women with breast cancer and BRCA gene have same prognosis at each stage as women who have breast cancer and do not have BRCA gene.

Classic syndromes associated with breast cancer

- Li–Fraumeni syndrome
    - p53 mutation
    - soft tissue sarcoma, osteosarcoma, breast cancer, brain tumors, leukemia
- Cowden's syndrome
    - *PTEN* mutation
    - breast, gastrointestinal, central nervous system, skin, eye, thyroid, genitourinary, bone cancers
- Peutz–Jeghers syndrome
    - *STK11* mutation
        - GI hamartomas, pigmented lesions,
        - Increased breast cancer risk
- hereditary nonpolyposis colon cancer
    - HNPCC mismatch repair gene
    - risk of endometrial, ovarian, colon, urinary, breast cancers increased
- ataxia-telangiectasia
    - DNA repair defect
      results in telangiectasias, cerebellar ataxia, increased risk of breast cancer

Stewart-Treves syndrome: may appear years after axillary lymph node dissection. Appears as purple nodules and ipsilateral arm swelling. Lymphangiosarcoma. Early metastasis to lungs.

Mondor's syndrome: thrombophlebitis of anterior chest wall following radical mastectomy. Presents as cord-like mass. Treat with NSAIDs.

IgA is found in breast milk

Breast Cancer and Pregnancy

- During the first and second trimesters, breast irradiation is contraindicated, and treatment includes MRM.
- May perform surgery in 2nd or 3rd trimester.
- NO RADIOSULFUR COLLOID in the pregnant patient.
- Chemo may be given after first trimester.

Inflammatory breast cancer

- Looks like abscess / breast infection so get a punch skin biopsy
- Histology demonstrates dermal lymphatic invasion
- Considered T4 lesion
- First do neoadjuvant therapy and AFTER do modified radical mastectomy

Tamoxifen is an estrogen receptor antagonist. Lesion must be estrogen receptor positive (ER +) for it to be useful. Older women are more often ER+. Tamoxifen decreases recurrence and mortality.

Bloody nipple discharge is usually due to intraductal papilloma, but still need to rule out cancer so do ductogram and excise duct.

Breast Cancer

- Risk in US = 1 in 8 women (12%)
- Screening decreases risk of death by approximately 25%
- If untreated, median survival 2 – 3 years
- Bone is most common site for metastasis
- Of all cases, 10% have negative mammogram and negative ultrasound
- Exam features may include nipple distortion / retraction, firm, fixed mass

Breast mass workup in adult

- do ultrasound and core needle biopsy.
    - If > 40, add bilateral mammograms.
    - If < 40 yoa, add bilateral mammograms if exam or ultrasound is either indeterminate of suspicious for cancer.
- If core needle biopsy is discordant with exam, non-diagnostic, or otherwise indeterminate perform excisional biopsy.
- If cyst: bloody cyst fluid on aspiration requires excisional biopsy. If fluid is clear & recurs after aspiration: requires excisional biopsy. If complex cyst: requires excisional biopsy. If solid component to cyst (at wall etc.) also needs tissue diagnosis.

Fine needle aspiration (FNA) gives only the cells involved in the lesion (cytology)

Core need biopsy gives cells and surrounding architecture

Mammogram

- Approximately 90% sensitive and specific for cancer
- More sensitive as patient ages because fat replaces dense breast tissue
- Findings consistent with cancer: irregular borders, spiculations, calcifications, architectural distortion

BI-RADS classification for mammogram findings

Category	Description	Recommendations
1	Negative	Routine screening
2	Benign	Routine screening
3	Probably benign	another mammogram in 3-6 months (rapid followup)
4	Suspicious	Obtain core needle biopsy (there's a 4a, 4b, & 4c subcategory with approximate cancer risk 15%, 35%, & 80% respectively)
5	Highly suggestive of cancer	Obtain core needle biopsy

BI-RADS 4 lesion with core needle biopsy that is...

- non-diagnostic, indeterminate or benign & non-concordant with mammogram
  obtain needle localized excisional biopsy
- benign and concordant with mammogram
  6 month followup
- malignant
  as per breast cancer treatment listed later

BI-RADS 5 lesion with core needle biopsy that is...

- anything other than malignancy
  needle localization excisional biopsy

- malignancy
  as per breast cancer treatment listed later

Mammographic screening

- Every 2-3 years after 40, then yearly after 50
- No mammogram in patients less than 40 unless high risk because < 40 has dense breast parenchyma making interpretation difficult
- High risk patients screening
  Mammogram 10 years prior to age at which youngest first degree relative was diagnosed with cancer

BRCA 1 is strongest risk factor for breast cancer

HER2/neu

- receptor positive cancer has worse prognosis stage for stage
- gene for this receptor is located on chromosome 17q
  part of epidermal growth factor receptor family.

- tyrosine kinase receptor
- Herceptin (trastuzumab, an antibody) blocks the HER2 / neu receptor

Screening MRI

- recommended for women with a known *BRCA* mutation
- those who have NOT undergone genetic testing but who do have a first degree relative with a known mutation or breast cancer prior to menopause
- women with > 20–25% lifetime risk for breast cancer
- and women who have a history of chest irradiation between 10 and 30 years of age.
- **Diagnostic** breast MRIs are indicated for new diagnoses of breast cancer, particularly in the presence of lobular cancer or dense breast tissue.

Breast cancer in males

- Worse prognosis in part because tends to present later
- Usually invasive ductal cancer
- Less than 1% of all breast cancer cases
- Increased pectoral muscle involvement
- Perform modified radical mastectomy

Ductal Carcinoma In Situ (DCIS)

- Breast cancer without invasion of the basement membrane.
- ductal epithelium proliferates resulting in comedo, cribiform, or papillary growth pattern.
- Precursor of ductal adenocarcinoma
- Five times increased risk in ipsilateral breast cancer.
- Usually affects women in their fifth to sixth decades.
- 15–20% of female and 5% of male breast cancer cases.
- Paget's disease of the breast is eczematous nipple change usually associated with underlying ipsilateral DCIS or invasive ductal cancer

Lobular Carcinoma In Situ (LCIS)

- Proliferation of duct lobules.
- Is NOT a precursor to ductal adenocarcinoma
- HOWEVER, LCIS is associated with a 30% risk of ductal adenocarcinoma in either breast. LCIS is a statistical marker for, but NOT precursor to, ductal adenocarcinoma
- Typically seen in premenopausal Caucasian women in the fifth decade.
- May be bilateral or multicentric. Commonly asymptomatic.
- Workup may or may not reveal adjacent calcifications on mammography.
- Treatment can include observation or bilateral prophylactic mastectomies with tamoxifen.

Ductal adenocarcinoma

- Most common cancer in females.
- Commonly presents in postmenopausal woman.
- Lifetime incidence is one in every 8–9 women.
- Classic presentation is painless, firm, & fixed mass. May also present as a firm axillary lymph node.
- Later may see skin retraction, nipple inversion, skin changes (ie, peau d'orange), bleeding, and ulceration.
- Can be associated with Paget's disease of the breast.
- Risk factors include

  Caucasian race, female gender, age > 50, early menarche, nulliparity, first pregnancy late in life, late menopause, history of breast cancer in first-degree relatives, prior breast cancer or atypical ductal hyperplasia, and presence of genetic syndrome (eg, BRCA1 or BRCA2)

- surgery attempts control of local disease (ie, lumpectomy or mastectomy) and evaluation of nodal disease.
    - Contraindications to breast-conserving surgery (lumpectomy and sentinel node biopsy) include
        - previous radiation to the affected breast
        - multicentric disease
        - large tumor relative to breast size that would result in an unacceptable cosmesis
        - high risk of local recurrence
    - Studies show no difference in overall or disease-free survival comparing lumpectomy with radiation to modified radical mastectomy
    - evaluation of nodal disease can be via sentinel lymph node biopsy (SLNB) or via axillary lymph node dissection.
    - Axillary dissection is indicated for
        - Positive SLNB
        - known lymph node positive disease based on preoperative FNA or clinical exam
        - presence of inflammatory breast cancer

Radiation therapy

- often used in combination with breast-conserving surgery
- Contraindicated in first and second trimesters of pregnancy
- Contraindicated in patients with a prior history of chest wall irradiation.
- decreases rate of local recurrence
- elderly patients with small hormone receptor positive tumors who are treated with adjuvant hormonal therapy may not require radiation therapy.

Chemotherapy

- Beneficial to all patients with high risk of relapse no matter what their nodal status may be.
- Can generally be withheld in patients with tumors < 1 cm and negative lymph nodes.
- Decreases recurrence rate by 30%.
- Anthracyclines in combination with taxanes such as paclitazel may also be effective.
- Combinations vary, but those containing anthracyclines are most effective
  For example: 5-fluorouracil [5-FU]-doxorubicin-cyclophosphamide or doxorubicin- cyclophosphamide

Hormonal therapy

- Reduces recurrence and mortality in patients with estrogen receptor positive tumors.
- helps prevent contralateral breast cancer in high-risk patients.
- Anastrozole
    - Aromatase inhibitor
    - may be used in postmenopausal women especially in those with contraindication to tamoxifen
    - May improve disease-free survival and risk of contralateral cancer compared to tamoxifen alone.
- Tamoxifen
    - Selective estrogen receptor modulator (SERM)
    - 20 mg/d for 5 years
    - Reduces risk of recurrent and contralateral breast cancer and improves overall and disease-free survival.
    - Also used for 1° prevention in high-risk groups where it decreases risk up to 50%.
    - Increased risk of endometrial cancer, stroke, and thromboembolic events.
    - Benefits also include increased bone density and decreased low-density lipoprotein (LDL) cholesterol.

- Trastuzumab
    - Monoclonal antibody to HER2/neu that may be used with HER2/neu positive breast cancer patients in both the adjuvant and metastatic setting.
      Side effects include cardiomyopathy

Lobular Carcinoma of the Breast

- About 10% of breast cancer cases.
- Presents as a poorly defined fibrotic mass
- More likely to be ER+/progesterone receptor positive (PR+), multicentric, and bilateral.
- Histology shows "indian filing" of lesion cells.

Cardiothoracic

Heart formation begins at third week of gestation.

Separation into atria starts with septum primum descending to close foramen primum.

In part of the septum primum, apoptosis occurs to create the foramen secundum and then a right-to-left shunt.

Remember, right to left shunt is correct direction in fetus because oxygenated blood from mother returns to R heart and need not go to lungs for oxygenation.

Septum secundum arises next to the septum primum. This creates foramen ovale (another location for right-to-left shunting).

When respiration begins, left-sided pressures increase and so the septum primum closes. The septum secundum is compressed and so the valve (fossa ovalis) closes.

Calcium binding drives contraction of smooth muscle.

Left main coronary branches into left anterior descending (LAD) and circumflex artery.

- LAD gives septal branches, which supply the interventricular septum, and diagonal branches, which supply the antero- lateral left ventricle (LV).
- Circumflex coronary artery provides marginal branches supplying the posterior and lateral LV.

Right coronary artery provides blood supply to the right ventricle, both the SA & AV nodes, & posterior inferior LV.

Starling curve describes the relationship between preload and contractility.

Cardiac output = (heart rate)(stroke volume)

Oxygen content of arterial blood = 1.39 (hemoglobin)(arterial 02 saturation) + (0.003)(Pa02)

Notice that oxygen delivery to tissues really depends on hemoglobin, 02 saturation, and cardiac output.

Oxygen content of venous blood = 1.39 (hemoglobin)(venous 02 saturation) + (0.003 Pv02)

Oxygen extraction ratio indicates 02 extracted from arterial blood. Therefore (oxygen content of arterial blood – oxygen content of venous blood) / (oxygen content of arterial blood) gives extraction ratio.

Oxygen delivery = (oxygen content of arterial blood)(cardiac output)

Dobutamine and Milrinone are ionotropes.

- Dobutamine works by stimulating beta 1 and beta 2 receptors. ("One heart, two lungs" reminds you that beta 1 receptors predominate in the heart and beta two predominate in the lungs.) With dobutamine: heart rate (HR) up, pulm artery wedge pressure (PAWP) down, cardiac index (CI) up, systemic vascular resistance (SVR) up down, mean arterial pressure (MAP) may be either up or down.
- Milrinone is a phosphodiesterase inhibitor. It also functions as a vasodilator. HR up, PAWP down, CI up, SVR down, MAP down.

Dopamine, norepinephrine, & epinephrine are mixed agents.

- Dopamine stimulates dopamine receptors, beta 1, beta 2 and alpha 1 receptors. HR increased, PAWP may be increased or decreased, CI up, SVR up or down, MAP up or down.
- Norepinephrine stimulates beta 1, beta 2, and alpha 1 receptors. HR increased, PAWP increased, CI up, SVR up, MAP up.
- Epinephrine stimulates beta 1, beta 2, and alpha 1 receptors. HR increased, PAWP increased or decreased, CI up, SVR up, MAP up.

Phenylephrine and Vasopressin are vasopressors

- Phenylephrine stimulates alpha 1 receptors. HR no change, PAWP increased, CI no change, SVR up, MAP up.
- Vasopressin stimulates V1 receptors in vascular smooth muscle to cause constriction. HR no change, PAWP no change, CI no change, SVR up, MAP up.

Nitroglycerine and nitroprusside are vasodilators

- Nitroglycerine causes smooth muscle relaxation. HR decreased, PAWP may decrease of no change, CI typically no change, SVR decreased, MAP decreased.
- Nitroprusside also causes smooth muscle relaxation. HR increased, PAWP decreased or no change, CI no change, SVR decreased, MAP decreased.

Ionotropes requiring chatecholamine stores: amrinone, milrinone, enoximone.

Amrinone is a phosphodiesterase inhibitor, activates cAMP system. Vasodilates and increases cardiac output. Utilizes endogenous catecholamines.

Cardiopulmonary bypass gives microemboli, creates hypoperfusion, and releases systemic inflammatory mediators. Related issues may be seen in every organ system.

- The heart may demonstrate stunning & reperfusion injury. Due to hypoperfusion & inflammatory mediators.
- The brain may show cognitive impairment & neuropsychiatric issues. Due to microemboli, hypoperfusion, symptoms, stroke, & inflammatory mediators.
- The lung may demonstrate hypoxia, edema, infarct, acute atelectasis, hypoperfusion, inflammatory respiratory distress syndrome (ARDS). Due to microemboli, inflammatory mediators, and capillary leak.
- The kidneys may show renal failure/insufficiency. Due to hemoglobin precipitation in tubules & hypoperfusion (leads to antithrombin III release).
- The liver may show transaminitis with hyperbilirubinemia. Due to microemboli, hypoperfusion, & inflammatory mediators.
- The pancreas may demonstrate clinically overt pancreatitis or mild chemical pancreatitis. Thought to be due to hypoperfusion or calcium administration.
- Blood may demonstrate Heparin-induced Thrombocytopenia (HIT) and coagulopathy. May be due to heparin administration, platelet dysfunction, clotting factor depletion, & fibrinolysis.

Right to left cardiac shunts give cyanosis, clubbing, polycythemia, & failure to thrive. Squatting down increases peripheral vascular resistance and ultimately left atrial pressure. So shunt decreases. Examples of R to L shunt:

- Truncus arteriosus
  - 22q11 deletion (Di George's syndrome). 80% mortality in first year of life if CHF noted. Often VSD present.
  - Cyanosis typically seen at birth, CHF within weeks, 02 sats approximately 80%.
  - Diuretics, digoxin, fluid restriction, afterload reduction.
  - Repair includes VSD repair, resection of PA from aorta (Ao), Ao repair, RV → PA conduit.
- Transposition of great vessels
  - Most common cyanotic CHD occurring in first week of life.
  - Death prevented by any shunt that mixes oxygenated and relatively deoxygenated blood such as PDA, ASD, VSD, or combinations of those.
  - Give PGE1. Balloon septoplasty (atrial) is palliative and repair consists of arterial switch operation with closure of septal defects and PDA.
- Tetraology of Fallot
- Will see a "BOOT" shaped heart = Big right ventricle, Overriding / overarching aorta, Open septum (Ventricular Septal Defect), Tiny valve (pulmonic)
- Most common cyanotic heart defect.
- More common in males.
- Associated with 22q11 defect (DiGeorge's Syndrome) and CATCH-22 syndrome.
- "Tet spells" are unpredictable hypoxic events caused by increased R to L flow through defect. Squatting down improves symptoms.
  - Treat spells with β-blocker, phenylephrine, morphine (morphine decreases peripheral vascular resistance).
- Blalock-Taussig shunt (systemic-to- pulmonary) is palliative not definitive.
- Operative repair includes right ventricular outflow tract enlargement, VSD repair.

Left to Right shunts cause CHF along with hepatomegaly, dyspnea, tachypnea etc. Examples:

- Atrial Septal Defect (ASD)
- Most common adult congenital defect.
- Secundum most common type. 1/1500 live births.
- More common in females.
- Paradoxical emboli, atrial arrhythmias, CHF, systolic ejection murmur (SEM) with fixed, split S2.
- Echo, catheterization, ECG.
- Treat with digoxin, diuretics, percutaneous repair. Repair all primum, CHF cases, & secundums that persist to school age.
- Ventricular Septal Defect (VSD)
- Most common congenital heart defect overall.
- Most close spontaneously by 6 months.
- pansystolic murmur
- Consider Eisenmenger's syndrome.
- Treat with digoxin, diuretics, catheter interventions. Repair at school age if still open, if PVR > 4–6 Woods units, or large defect.
- Patent Ductus Arteriosus
- Common in premature infants.
- Failure to thrive, dyspnea, tachycardia, arrhythmias, continuous machine-like murmur.
- Indomethacin closes PDA. PGE2 keeps open. Operative ligation if no response to meds.

Other congenital cardiac defects:

- Total anomalous pulmonary venous return
- More common in males. PDA present for mixing.
- Severe cyanosis, RV heave, fixed, split S2, + S3.
- CXR has snowman sign
- PGE1 is palliative
- Operative repair includes rerouting of pulmonary veins.
- Aortic coarctation
- Most common in Caucasian males.
- Associated with Turner's (XO) syndrome, bicuspid aortic valve.
- Discrepancy in BP between right/left arms and upper/ lower extremities
- CXR with rib notching and "3 sign", catheterization, echo.

Valve replacement options for acquired valvular heart disease:

- Mechanical (eg, St. Jude): Most durable. **Requires anticoagulation (eg warfarin) therapy**.
- Bioprosthetic (eg, porcine allograft, bovine pericardium): Less durable. Does not require anticoagulation always.
- Cadaveric (eg, homograft): Least durable. Does not require anticoagulation.
- Consider tissue valves (shorter lasting as above, but no anti coag needed) in patients who may become pregnant, have contraindication to coumadin; also used for all tricuspid replacements

Aortic stenosis is the most common acquired valvular heart disease.

Mitral stenosis is associated with rheumatic fever.

Bypass conduit durability: LIMA > saphenous vein > radial artery

Idiopathic hypertrophic subaortic stenosis (IHSS) is treated with septal resection, and is leading cause of sudden death in children and adolescents. Demonstrates hypertrophic typically of interventricular septum resulting in obstruction of left ventricular outflow tract.

Cardiac myxoma is most common primary tumor of the heart.

- Typically affects women in the third to sixth decade of life.
- Usually involve the left atrium.
- Risk is emboli and atrial outflow obstruction.
- Presents like mitral stenosis. Diagnose with echo.
- Treatment is resection.

Intra Aortic Balloon Pump (IABP): augments diastolic coronary blood flow and reduces afterload by inflating during diastole. Inflates 40 msec before T wave, deflates with p wave.

Levels where structures enter / leave through diaphragm

- T8 Vena Cava
- T10 Esophagus (and vagi)
- T12 Thoracic duct and aorta

Type I alveoli: functional gas exchange

Type II: produce surfactant (decrease surface tension). These are 1% of alveoli

Classify lung cancer as non small cell (80% of cases) and small cell cancer (20% of cases).

Non-small cell class includes adenocarcinoma, squamous cell cancer, etc.

Adenocarcinoma is most common lung cancer in US

Squamous cell lung cancer associated with PTH-like substance

Small cell lung CA associated with ACTH and ADH

T1: < 3cm, T2 > 3cm, T3 invasion of chest wall, pericardium, diaphragm, < 2 cm from carina; T4 = unresectable = into mediastinum, heart, great vessel, esophagus, trachea, vertebrae, effusion

N1: ipsi hilar nodes; N2: ipsi mediastinal; N3 = unresectable = contralateral or scalene or subclavian nodes

CT abdomen and chest is single best test for determining T and N status

PET scan is single best test for determining M (metastasis) status

Mediastinoscopy is used to obtain tissue diagnosis on lesions that are centrally located and demonstrate mediastinal adenopathy > 0.8cm or > 1.0cm (subcarinal position).

- If tissue from mediastinal nodes is positive for cancer then tumor can not be resected.
- Can NOT assess AP (aorto-pulmonary) window nodes. For that you need the...

Chamberlain procedure (performed via anterior thoracotomy or parasternal mediastinotomy). Procedure evaluates AP window nodes as mediastinoscopy can not evaluate those. Incision may be made via left 2nd rib cartilage.

Bronchoscopy may be performed to check for airway invasion of lesion.

Stage 1: T1-2N0; II: T2N1; IIIa up to T3 or N2; IIIb unresectable T4 or N3; IV: M1 NB: Left lung can drain to right mediastinum (remember left to right just like reading)

- Stage I and II: Anatomic resection (lobectomy) has improved survival over wedge resection. May substitute sleeve resection (if bronchial margin cannot unable to be obtained via lobectomy) or pneumonectomy (large, centrally located tumors or bulky, extracapsular N1 nodal spread). Tumors involving chest wall / diaphragm removed en bloc. Consider limited surgical resection (eg wedge resection) or radiotherapy for poor operative candidates.
- Stage III (locoregionally advanced disease): In patients with limited node involvement or accessible tumors, surgical resection continues to play a role. In stage **IIIA patients, cisplatin-based neoadjuvant chemotherapy followed by surgical resection is the standard.** Stage IIIB patients are not generally operative candidates (except for tumors involving the SVC, carina, or vertebral bodies with N0 or N1 dis- ease). Most locoregionally advanced cases are treated with cisplatin-based chemoradiation (concurrent or sequential).
- Stage IV (metastatic disease): Chemotherapy is the mainstay. Select patients with a single brain metastasis may be candidates for excision of both the 1° and metastatic tumor.

Diagnosis of primary lung cancer

- begins with a thorough history and physical exam. The major risk factors are smoking and asbestos exposure (in smokers).
- Clinically, patients may present with cough, hemoptysis, chest pain, dyspnea, pleural effusion, clubbing, hoarseness, or remain asymptomatic.
- Diagnostic studies should begin with chest x-rays.
- Suspicious lesions should be followed up with a CT scan to assess local spread and to check for metastases. The adrenal glands and liver should be included in the thoracic CT.

- Histological diagnosis should be attempted by sputum cytology, bronchoscopy, bronchial biopsy, brushings or washings, or by percutaneous transthoracic needle biopsy.
- Mediastinoscopy is helpful in determining hilar involvement in patients with nodes larger than 1 cm in the hilum as seen on CT scan.
- Bone scans and brain CT are indicated studies in symptomatic patients.
- The usual signs of inoperability include:
  - Bloody pleural effusion
  - Horner's syndrome
  - Vocal cord paralysis
  - Phrenic nerve paralysis
  - Superior vena cava syndrome
  - Distant mets

Non-small cell CA chemotherapy (stage II or greater) is carboplatinin, Taxol

Small cell lung CA chemotherapy is cisplatin, etoposide

In lung cancer cases, patients need to be both **resectable** (no N2, N3, or M disease) and **operable** (*ie* have appropriate FEV1 and DLCO values)

Pre-thoracotomy PFTs & procedure patient can tolerate. (DLCO and FEV1 cut-offs for operability)...

- FEV1 > 2L for pneumonectomy
- FEV1 > 1L for lobectomy
- FEV1 > 0.6L for wedge resection
- Need postop predicted FEV1 > 40% postop value (typically 0.8L)
  Best predictor of postop complications
- Need DLCO > 40% predicted postop value (typically > 10)

Thymoma: indication for resection Resecting thymus (even if no thymoma) in myasthenia gravis improves 90% (10% of m.g. have thymomas)

Popcorn lesion on CXR is classically a *hamartoma* Thoracic outlet syndrome rarely involves artery or vein (1-3%), generally *ulnar* n paresthesias

Spontaneous PTX 10:1 male predilection; 50% recur then 75% of those again. Thoracoscopy for 2nd or cont air leak

Post MI VSD presents day 2-7; 2% of MI's; pan-systolic murmur SVC syndrome: 90% due to lung CA; Rx with XRT

Takayasu arteritis: young female, involves thoracic and abdominal aorta and PA. Angiogram diagnoses.

Rheumatic fever leads to *mitral stenosis*; see regurg with MI or valve degeneration

Chylothorax (non-iatrogenic) usually due to posterior mediastinal tumor (75% lymphoma). XRT may help. Thoracic duct injury: treat with drainage/NPO x 2 wks; if not resolved then R thoracotomy, ligate duct

Thoracic duct enters chest on R with Aorta at T12, crosses to left at T4, joins IJ/Subclavian junction

Thoracic aorta aneuryms, operate for > 6 cm, symptomatic

Aortic Dissection: Stanford type A -> involves ascending aorta, must operate; Stanford type B does not involve ascending aorta. Medical management.

CAD: leading killer in U.S. (2x Cancer)

CABG indications: intractable symptoms, > 50% left main, triple vessel dis, or 70% LAD + 1 other vessel

Angioplasty: 20% restenosis by 1 yr; vein graft 5 yr patency 80%; IMA graft approximately 95% patency at 20 yrs

VSD: as mentioned #1 cardiac congenital defect, 50% close on their own, OR if symptomatic or failure to thrive

PDA: close all those that *indomethacin* does not at 6 months of age

Defects in Endocardial Cushion Development

- Most common (60-70%): Complete AV Septal defect, presence of both atrial and ventricular septal defects with a common AV valve
- must correct prior to pulmonary hypertension and pulmonary cardiac failure.

Neuroblastoma occurs in the posterior mediastinum as a mediastinal mass in the pediatric population.

Determination of myocardial oxygen consumption/energy expenditure:

Myocardial oxygen extraction is 60%; consumption increases in demand or poor oxygenation.

Heart gets blood during diastole.

Oxygen extraction ratio = (arterial oxy - venous oxygen)/arterial oxygen.

Atrial naturetic peptide: released by atrial stretching and CNS injury and causes diuresis by naturesis (sodium loss in urine)

Facts about MI

- Pulmonary Artery Catheter in Acute MI demonstrates increased pressures because end diastolic volume is increased. There is also increased systemic vascular resistance and decreased cardiac output.
- Pan systolic murmur after MI is VSD or papillary muscle necrosis and mitral regurgitation.
- Left Internal Mammary Artery is the best conduit for Coronary Artery Bypass grafts
- Hypertrophic subaortic stenosis should be managed with ACE inhibitors, beta blockade and decreasing myocardial demand. Do not use dopamine in this disease because it increases myocardial demand.
- Rx cardiogenic shock first treat disease and second give dobutamine.

Signs of pericardial tamponade include muffled heart sounds, decreased blood pressure, and collapsed right atrium on echo.

Etiology of death in patients with heart transplants is atherosclerosis with thrombosis of grafts. Grafts are denervated so these MIs cases typically do not include pain.

Treatment of SVC syndrome: Balloon angioplasty/ stent/ catheter lysis/ Treat underlying malignancy.

Aortic insufficiency causes angina because of diastolic blood flow to the coronaries.

Aortic Dissection

- Type A Involves ascending aorta ("Affects Ascending Aorta And Arch"). Must be repaired. 60% of cases. May result in aortic valve incompetence and / or rupture into pericardial sac with tamponade.
- Type B Descending aorta ("Begins Beyond Brachiocephalic vessels"). Treatment is medical management. Distal to L subclavian takeoff.

Heme-oxy dissociation curve shifts to the right (offloading 02 is easier, onloading is tougher) with an increase in EVERYTHING **EXCEPT pH and carbon monoxide**. So...

- Curve shifts to the right with increased
- 2,3 DPG
- temperature
- carbon dioxide
- hydrogen ions (opposite shift from pH because of how pH is calculated)

Paraneoplastic syndromes with associated cancers

- Adenocarcinoma
  Hypertrophic periostitis seen in fibula, tibia, radius, metacarpals, & metatarsals. May see clubbing & osteoarthropathy.

- Squamous cell lung cancer & thymoma
  - Eaton-Lambert
    Caused by antibodies against Ca2+ channels. Syndrome causes weakness that improves with repeated movement. Neostigmine is NOT effective.

  - SIADH
    High urine osmolarity despite low serum osmolarity

  - Cushing's syndrome
    Patients fail dexamethasone suppression test

  - Squamous cell cancer
    - Hypercalcemia
      Increased calcium due to parathyroid related peptide (PTHrP).

Pancoast tumor is a tumor at superior sulcus that affects the sympathetic trunk & brachial plexus causing anhydrosis, ptosis, and miosis.

NB: Pancoast tumor involves sympathetic chain (Horner's syndrome) and/or *ulnar* nerve

Mesothelioma: often called most malignant lung cancer. Related to asbestos exposure. Characterized by locally aggressive invasion, nodal invasion, and distant metastases. All common at time of diagnosis.

SVC syndrome is treated with emergent Xray therapy if due to cancer

Coin shaped lesion on imaging...

- About 10% are malignant (of all-comers)
- Most common
    - lesion is granuloma
    - tumor is hamartoma
    - cancer is adenocarcinoma
- For patients < 50, < 5% are malignant
- But for patients aged > 50, 50% are malignant
- No growth in 2 years, and smooth contour suggests benign disease.
- If suspicious for any reason, will require guided biopsy or wedge resection

Carcinoid of lung is a neuroendocrine tumor that is typically centrally located. About half of patients demonstrate symptoms such as cough or hemoptysis. Minority of patients (5%) have metastases when diagnosed. If positive nodes or > 3cm tumor, probability of recurrence is significantly increased.

Most common benign lung tumor in adults is hamartoma. Diagnosis may be made on CT where calcifications and "popcorn lesion" may be visible. Does not require resection. Re-CT in 6 months to confirm.

Transplantation

CD-4 (T Helper cell) interacts with antigen-presentation via MHC II on macrophages (Kupfer cells in liver) to proliferate and produce IL-2. Remember which CD4 with which MHC via "4 times 2 equals 8", *eg* CD4 with MHC 2 and CD8 with MHC I. (8 times 1 equals one.) So MHC class times CD class always equals 8.

CD8 cells (Cytotoxic T cells) activated by IL-2 and interact with MHC I (present on all nucleated cells). This results in damage to transplanted organ / rejection.

Macrophages release IL-1 which goes to hypothalamus and causes fever.

Neutrophils bind to selectins (glycoproteins) which are found on endothelium. P selectin is on platelets and endothelial cells. E selectin is on endothelium. L selectin is on lymphocytes. These allow neutrophil "rolling".

Integrins bind to ICAM on endothelial cell. They are on neutrophil. Activated by chemokines and help with adhesion to endothelium. These allow neutrophil "firm adherence".

IgA is common immuglobulin in the gut. Found typically in Peyer's Patches.

Graft vs host disease is T cell mediated.

Hyperacute rejection is due to pre-formed antibodies (avoided by not transplanting when crossmatch is positive). Thymoglobulin & now desensitization protocols (plasmapheresis and IVIG) also help avoid this.

Acute rejection due to foreign MHC antigens from graft cells. Bx shows lymphocytic infiltrate. Treat with steroid bolus ("if you give a damn, give a gram [of methylpred]") or with OKT3

Chronic rejection results in gradual loss of blood supply. No good treatment

Immunosuppression is largely cellular and not humoral system, therefore viral risk > bacterial

See increased CA (skin, leukemia, lymphoma, cervical)
CMV is #1 virus post-transplant

Azathioprine: 6MP (mercapto purine) derivative, purine analog that acts as an antimetabolite, decr DNA synthesis

Mycophenolate (MMF, aka cellcept): blocks purine synthesis to decrease T and B cell proliferation as an inosine monophosphate dehydrogenase inhibitor. Remember that WBCs lack a purine salvage pathway. So without ability to make new DNA (no adenine and guanine [purines] so no DNA) and without ability to salvage purines, T and B cells can not proliferate. Azathioprine has similar mechanism. Side effects include myelosuppression and GI intolerance.

Cyclosporine: ultimately inhibits mRNA encoding IL-2. Binds cyclophilin protein and inhibits calcineurin. Undergoes hepatic metabolism and biliary excretion. Has enterohepatic circulation. Adverse effects of cyclosporine include hirsutism, neurotoxicities, hyperkalemia, nephrotoxicity and hepatotoxicity. The most frequent toxic effects are nephrotoxicity, hypertension and tremors.

Tacrolimus aka FK506: Calcineurin inhibitor. More potent than cyclosporine & blocks IL-2 expression/production from T cells.

Sirolimus (rapamycin) inhibits mTOR (TOR stands for Target of Rapamycin). Inhibits T and B cell response to IL-2. Side effect is interstitial lung disease. NOT nephrotoxic.

Prednisone works in cell nucleus to inhibit mRNA. Blocks creation of IL-2.

Thymoglobulin (aka "thymo" or ATG for anti-thymocyte globulin): ATGAM if isolated from horses, "thymo" if isolated from rabbits. Polyclonal antibodies against CD2, CD3, & CD4. Side effects include cytokine release syndrome (pulmonary edema, chills, shock, fever, kidney damage). Premedicate with steroids and benadryl prior to administration.

OKT3, a monoclonal antibody, used to treat rejection

Biliary stricture post liver transplant? Check hepatic artery flow, may be due to ischemia

Ureteral stricture post-renal transplant (months)? Check for BK virus.

#1 cause of oliguria s/p renal transplant is ATN

Cardiac transplant: 84% 1 yr survival

Liver transplant: 70% 1 yr graft survival

Major Histocompatibility Complex in humans is called HLA (Human Leukocyte Antigen)

HLA-A, -B, and -DR (Human Leukocyte Antigen) are the most significant in donor and recipient matching. HLA-A, -B, and -D pairs are usually inherited together. Because of this, there are four possible combinations for child to inherit. One of two versions A, B & D from one parent and one of two versions from another because A, B & D stick together. So four combinations possible.

HLA A, B & C = Class I (MHC I)

HLA D, DQ & DR / DW = Class 2 (MHC II)

HLA-DR is the most important overall

ABO blood compatibility is typically required for all transplants (except liver)

- Type O is universal donor
- Type AB is universal recipient

Cross-match

- tests for preformed antibodies in recipient to the donor organ by mixing recipient serum with donor lymphocytes.
- Positive if these antibodies are present, it is considered positive

If positive, hyperacute rejection would likely occur with transplant

Panel reactive antibody (PRA)

- Technique similar to cross-match
- detects preformed recipient antibodies using a panel of cells with different HLAs.
- Returns a percentage of cells that the recipient serum reacts with
- PRA > 50% indicates increased risk of hyperacute rejection and is a contraindication to transplant
- Previous cadaveric bone graft, transfusions, pregnancy, transplant, and autoimmune diseases increase PRA

Cell mediated immunity is T cell mediated. Humoral immunity is B cell mediated. Some rejection episodes include both T cell mediated and B cell mediated responses. IVIG treats humoral rejection. Cell mediated rejection episodes are usually treated with steroids.

Treat mild rejection with pulse steroids

Treat severe rejection with steroid and antibody therapy (thymoglobulin) although there are many options.

Most common malignancy following any is skin cancer (squamous cell CA #1)

Post-transplant lympho-proliferative disorder is Epstein Barr virus related and is next most common malignancy post transplant following squamous cell cancer. May present as abdominal mass, adenopathy, +/- bowel obstruction. Treatment includes reduction of immunosuppression & rituximab (anti-CD20 antibody; decreases B cells). XRT and chemotherapy are also options for aggressive lesions.

Ability to tolerate cold ischemia varies among different organs. Kidney = 36–40 hours. Pancreas up to 24 hours. Liver: 16 hours. Heart/Lung: Up to 6 hours. Tolerable cold ischemic time is related to the metabolic activity of the tissue involved. More activity means less cold ischemic time available.

Most common cause of external ureteral compression in kidney transplant is lymphocele. Occurs approximately three weeks post transplant. Attempt perc drainage and if fails open peritoneum over collection (peritoneal window) to allow drainage.

Macrosteatosis > 50% gives 50% risk liver will not function if transplanted. Fat content of potential liver for transplant is predictive of non-function.

Early HAT (hepatic artery thrombosis) of transplanted liver typically requires emergent re-transplant owing to fulminant hepatic failure.

HAT after early post-op period may result in bile leak. Late HAT results in biliary strictures and / or abscess.

Timing is very useful to determine post-transplant infections: Candida infection, parasitic infections, and typical post op bacterial infections may occur early (first month) along with Hep B / C infection of allograft. CMV typically occurs after first month. Aspergillus and other potential fungal infections also occur later.

Trauma

Trauma deaths occur in three peaks post injury:

- 0-30 minutes is first peak and is typically owing to catastrophic injuries. Patients are typically not salvageable.
- 30 minutes – 4 hours is second peak. 50% due to traumatic brain injury (TBI) and 50% due to bleeding. Approximately 30% of deaths in this group occur during "golden hour".
- Days to weeks is third peak. Typically due to long term issues such as sepsis and multisystem organ failure.

"GCS < 8 then intubate"

#1 cause of preventable blunt trauma death is missed intra-abdominal injury

Types of shock

- Hypovolemic
  - Mechanism is decreased preload
  - Heart rate (HR) is typically elevated
  - Cardiac output (CO) down
  - Pallor, feet are cool
  - Give volume
- Cardiogenic
  - Mechanism is decreased contractility
  - HR is elevated
  - CO decreased
  - Only type with + jugular venous distension (JVD)
  - Dobutamine, levophed
- Septic
  - Mechanism is decreased afterload
  - HR is elevated
  - CO elevated
  - May be febrile, may have warm extremities
  - Source control, volume, levophed +/- vasopressin
- Neurogenic
  - Mechanism is decreased afterload
  - HR is elevated
  - CO is elevated
  - Spine fracture, paraplegia
  - volume, phenylephrine

FYI: the "zones" for abdominal trauma are for BLUNT trauma situations. For penetrating trauma, abdominal zones are not used for decision making. (There is no "zone 3 injury from gunshot wound" or "zone 2 injury with hematoma near kidney from gunshot wound".)

Classes of hemorrhage

- Class 1
  - Blood loss < 750 mL
  - HR normal
  - Pulse pressure normal
  - Blood pressure normal
  - Mental status normal
  - Resuscitation is crystalloid volume
- Class 2
  - Blood loss 750 mL to 1.5L (15-30% total blood volume)
  - HR > 100
  - Pulse pressure decreased
  - Blood pressure normal
  - Mental status = anxious
  - Resuscitation is crystalloid volume
- Class 3
  - Blood loss 1.5-2L (30-40%)
  - HR > 120
  - Pulse pressure decreased
  - Blood pressure decreased
  - Mental status confused
  - Resuscitation crystalloid and blood
- Class 4
  - Blood loss > 2 L
  - HR > 140
  - Pulse pressure decreased
  - Blood pressure decreased
  - Mental status lethargic
  - Resuscitation is crystalloid and blood

Notice blood pressure is ok until class 3 shock aka > 30% blood volume lost (!)

Initial fluid bolus in infants is 20mL/kg

Damage control surgery for trauma patients

- Stop bleeding and control contamination.
- Also used sometimes for emergency general surgery patients to decrease risk for post op abdominal compartment syndrome/improve physiology before subjecting to lengthy case.)
- Delay definitive repair until physiology (acidosis/hypothermia/hypocalcemia) improved / patient stabilized & coagulopathy corrected
- Resuscitate with RBCs to FFP to platelets in 1:1:1 ratio
- Typically leave abdomen open with temporary negative pressure dressing
- Permissive hypotension is an option except if patient may have a traumatic brain injury, in which case keep SBP > 90.

Cardiac tamponade on echo: may see collapsed left or right atrium. On inspiration L ventricle gets small and R gets big. Tapped blood does not clot. Good idea to leave drain in place if you've tapped off a tamponade or performed subxiphoid window. Hypotension is due to decreased diastolic filling.

Diagnostic Peritoneal Lavage

- Indication is hypotensive (SBP < 90) patient with blunt trauma
- Positive if obvious food or gross blood noted
- Perform via supra-umbilical incision if obvious or suspected pelvic fractures
- Rapid interpretation of DPL results: "newspaper test" = if you can read the newspaper through the fluid returned from abdomen (eg it's fairly clear / only blood tinged), DPL is negative
- Strict criteria for + DPL = > 10mL blood, > 100,000 RBCs / mL, bile, bacteria, > 500 WBCs / mL
- DPL misses retroperitoneal injuries
- Patient generally needs laparotomy if + DPL

FAST (Focused Abdominal Sonogram for Trauma)

- Examiner dependent
- Need approximately 250mL (one soda can) of free fluid / blood in abdomen to be seen on ultrasound
- Misses retroperitoneal injuries
- Checks for fluid in multiple views, most sensitive view is space between liver and R kidney (Morrison's pouch)
- + FAST in hypotensive patient generally means laparotomy required

Indications for thoracotomy (in OR)

- 1500mL out on initial chest tube placement or > 200mL / hour for 4 hours. (Threshold for amount over 4 hours is different from different sources.)
- Instability
- Incompletely drained hemothorax despite 2 good tubes
    - Need to drain blood in chest within 48 hours to prevent trapped lung with fibrous peel and infected hemothorax
    - Retained hemothorax is the most important risk factor for empyema

ED thoracotomy indications

- Should be used very selectively in blunt trauma patients. Indications vary per different sources. Some include use ONLY if loss of vital signs in ER.
- For penetrating trauma, loss of vitals immediately prior to ER arrival or in ER are more common indications
- Standard ED thoracotomy moves
    - Open pericardium anterior to phrenic nerve, insert digits and bluntly open rest of pericardium to preserve phrenic
    - Mainstem ET tube intentionally into R mainstem bronchus to allow L lung to be more easily manipulated
    - Feel for OGT position to identify location of esophagus and to help determine location of aorta.
    - Pulmonary hilar twist may be required if hilar injury, devastating lung injury
    - Cross clamp aorta low (near diaphragm) to avoid Artery of Adamkiewicz (Anterior spinal artery) and help prevent post procedure neuro deficits

Type O blood is universal donor. Contains no A or B antigens on cells. Often used during severe trauma situations. Rh negative blood ("O negative") typically for females who are of childbearing age or pre-pubescent. Rh positive ("O positive") is acceptable for males.

Catecholamine response to injury is maximal at 24-48 hours
Also see increased ADH, increased ACTH (which increases cortisol and aldosterone). Many other hormones such as T4 (thyroxin) from thyroid gland are NOT involved.

Spleen injury

- OPSI (Overwhelming Post Splenectomy Infection)
    - Greatest incidence is late post-splenectomy (years later) and NOT in first few days / weeks post op
    - Overall, RARE complication
    - Immunizations post-splenectomy are to protect against encapsulated organisms: H flu, N meningiditis, pneumococcus. Need pneumovax booster years post op.
- Unstable patients go to OR for splenectomy. Do not attempt splenic salvage with angioembolization
- Higher the injury grade in blunt trauma, more likely to fail non-op management.
- Complete healing takes about 5-6 weeks

Splenectomy (some facts related to trauma and related to elective splenectomy...)

- *tuftsin, properidin, fibronectin* (non-specific opsonins) no longer present
- decreased IgM production
- Approximately 10% of patients have an accessory spleen
- Splenectomy helps *all* patients with hereditary spherocytosis (anemia and jaundice remit)
  helps 80% of patients w/ITP
- Do not do splenectomy for patients with TTP (low plts, hemolytic anemia, neuro changes). Treatment is plasmapheresis

Epidural hematoma

- Lens shaped ("lenticular") appearance on head CT
- Lacerated middle meningeal artery
- Although "lucid interval" is classic presentation, many patients with epidural do NOT have that (although some do)
- Indications for OR include significant neuro deficit or shift (mass effect) > 5mm

Subdural hematoma

- Indications for procedure include mass effect > 1 cm or significant neuro changes
- Tearing of bridging veins that cross subdural space

Diffuse Axonal Injury (DAI)

- Initial head CT commonly does not show abnormality
- Treatment is supportive
- Prognosis and neuro outcome depend high on location of DAI in brain
- Owing to shearing of neurons as gray and white matter shear during rotation. This is because of the difference in mass of gray versus white matter. So when rotation occurs, different velocity during rotation causes shearing.

Intra Cranial Pressure (ICP) monitors are indicated for...

- GCS < 8
- Suspected ICP elevation
- Inability to monitor clinical exam (seen with intubated patients) in patients with severe or moderate head injury

Cerebral Perfusion Pressure (CPP)

- MAP – ICP = CPP ("mean arterial pressure minus intra-cranial pressure is cerebral perfusion pressure").
  Low CPP yields additional secondary brain trauma (< 60 or 70 depending on source and clinical situation)
- MAP = (2/3)(diastolic blood pressure) + (1/3)(systolic blood pressure)
- Note that therefore most of your average blood pressure is attributable to diastolic blood pressure
- On CT, certain findings correlate with elevate ICP
  - Decreased ventricle size
  - Loss of sulci
  - Loss of cisterns

ICP > 20 requires rapid treatment, also keep CPP > 60. Remember ICP typically peaks 48-72 hours after injury. Bradycardia is a sign of impending herniation and Cushing's triad is bradycardia, hypertension, and low respiratory rate. Treatments for ICP elevation include:

- Head of Bed (HOB) elevation
- Hyperventilation (to C02 values in low 30s range)
  Effect is transient and hyperventilation to lower values may cause vasoconstriction and decreased D02
- Achieve serum Na+ 140-150 and serum osmolarity 295-310
  May utilize 3% NS
- Pentobarbital (barbiturate) coma
  Requires EEG monitoring at most centers as well as an aggressive bowel regimen owing to ileus
- Mannitol
- Craniotomy
- Keppra / Dilantin (usually as an adjunct rather than primary treatment)
- Dilated / "blown" pupil related to oculomotor nerve (cranial nerve 3) pressure from temporal lobe. Remember to address hypotension if present *prior* to other interventions or imaging.

Basilar skull fractures

- Anterior fossa fracture may give raccoon eyes
- May see hemotympanum and CSF via nose
- Middle fossa fracture may give cranial nerve 7 injury (facial fracture) and Battle's sign

Temporal skull fractures may be associated with facial nerve injury at geniculate ganglion level (most common site of facial nerve injury). Most common cause of facial nerve injury is temporal bone fracture.

Skull fractures with significant depression (> 1cm), contamination, or continued CSF despite conservative therapy require surgical treatment. Most skull fractures do not require operative intervention.

Release tissue thromboplastin makes some patients demonstrate coagulopathy after brain injury.

Jefferson fracture is C1 burst fracture and is usually caused by axial loading.

Hangman's fracture is a type of C2 fracture and is usually caused by extension

C2 odontoid fractures can be separated into 3 types

- Type 2 is at base of dens process and is unstable. Typically requires halo or fusion.
- Type 3 is also unstable. Requires halo or fusion. Extends into vertebrae.
- Type 1 is a stable fracture and is above base of dens process.

Vertebral artery injury: ligate or embolize. Sequelae are unusual. Common carotid bleeding, in contrast, carries approximately 20% stroke rate with unilateral ligation.

All penetrating neck trauma with hard signs (eg shock, expanding hematoma, airway loss, etc.) need operative exploration.

Neck zones

- Whether blunt or penetrating trauma, if hard signs all need exploration.
- If blunt trauma and symptomatic: neck CT scan
- If penetrating and no hard signs, controversial. In general, see beneath. By zone...
- I = below cricoid
  Injury evaluations commonly require angio, bronchoscopy, and esophagoscopy / barium swallow

- II = cricoid to angle of jaw
  Easiest to explore in OR. Non-operative evaluation (evaluate all three "tubes" in the neck with imaging / EGD) and operative evaluation consider to have equivalent missed injury rate

- III = jaw to skull
  Need angiography and laryngoscopy

Esophageal injury

- Drain esophageal and hypopharyngeal repairs because approx. 20% leak rate
- If unusure regarding presence of esophageal injury in neck, leave drain
- This is a challenging injury to identify in the neck (thus rule regarding drainage as above). Some sources say this is the most difficult neck injury to find.
  - Contained injuries may be observed
  - Non-contained injuries
    - With extensive contamination or extensive injuries
      - Chest: place chest tubes to drain injury and create spit fistula in neck. Therefore usually requires esophagectomy owing to intentional loss of esophageal continuity.
        - Upper 2/3 of esophagus in thorax is approached via R thoracotomy
        - Lower 1/3 of esophagus is approached via L thoracotomy
      - Neck: place drains (extensive drainage) and will eventually heal

Tracheal injuries: ET tube placed beyond level of injury for approximately 5 days usually allows this area to heal

Bronchial tree injury

Sucking chest wounds

- Chest tube may show continuous air leak
- Large pneumomediastinum may be present
- Oxygenation may worsen after chest tube placed, one of very few indications to clamp a chest tube
- More common on the right
- Intubate patient with mainstem ETT placed on opposite side of injury
- 90% are within one cm of carina and therefore bronchoscopy is usually diagnostic
- repair if
  - large leak and respiratory compromise
  - more than 2 weeks with persistent air leak
  - lung will not fully inflate
  - injury greater than 1/3 of tracheal diameter

- Injury needs to be large (2/3 diameter of trachea) to be clinically significant
- Make one-way valve with dressing over hole on chest tapped on three sides

Diaphragm injury

- Despite newer evidence that says diaphragm injuries on R and L are of similar incidence, the test answer and "fact" remains that injuries are more common on the LEFT from blunt trauma and that the liver "blocks" on the right so less injuries there
  Diaphragm rupture from blunt trauma: classic teaching is 8:1 left side vs. right side
- Sometimes diagnosed with xray in trauma bay where OGT goes down into abdomen and then coils back into chest
- Transabdominal approach generally easier if < 1 week
- May cause tachycardia
- Chest approach if > 1 week (adhesions have formed in abdomen)
- May require PTFE mesh for repair

Aortic transection

- Approximately ½ die in the field, of the ½ that make it to the hospital, approximately ½ die in 6 hours if untreated
- Patients with first and second rib fractures are at high risk for aortic transection. Rule them out for it.
- Wide mediastinum is the best xray indicator of aortic injury, but unfortunately is also seen in many patients who don't have aortic injury. Other signs seem sometimes include first / second rib fractures, apical capping, loss of AP window, tracheal deviation (toward the right) but all of these are poor tests and of them wide mediastinum is probably the only generally useful one. And as mentioned even that one is generally weak.
- Overall CXR is NORMAL in 5% with aortic tears; therefore additional imaging (CT) is important
- Tear is at ligamentum arteriosum (distal to subclavian takeoff)
- Covered stent endograft is the repair for the majority of injuries (distal injuries only)
- Address other life threatening injuries first (eg unstable with positive DPL, address abdomen first) because patients who have lived with aortic transection from blunt trauma to make it to the hospital would die from their abdominal bleeding before their aortic injury
- Traumatic brain injury with ICH is a contraindication to operative repair (need for bypass)

Sternal fracture patients are at high risk for cardiac contusion.

Flail chest

- 2 or more consecutive ribs broken in 2 or more segments
- look for underlying pulmonary contusion

Penetrating injury to the chest

- the "box' = space bounded by clavicles, nipples, xiphoid process
- inside the box: typically require bronch, esophagoscopy, barium swallow, & pericardial window
  pericardial window: if blood, needs median sternotomy. Leave drain in pericardial sac after window. Go to OR.
- often also require angio for low zone 1 neck injuries and high chest trauma
- outside the box: remember, if intubation, consider chest tube placement even if no pneumothorax or hemothorax visible
- penetrating injuries below nipple but antero-medial to mid-axillary line
  - need laparotomy or laparoscopy
  - at times same workup as penetrating box injury (varies with specific location)

Laryngeal fractures

- Airway emergency
- May have crepitus and other hard signs
- Secure airway on emergent basis, often in ER. May require surgical airway.

Pelvic Trauma

- Unstable with pelvic fractures, negative DPL, and no other signs of blood loss: place t-pod, use bedsheet with clamps, or otherwise stabilize pelvis and go to angio for embolization
- Unstable pelvic fractures like open book fractures are at high risk for genitourinary and abdominal injuries
- Remember that severe pelvic trauma requires endoscopic evaluation of rectum and retrograde cystogram.
  - Posterior pelvic fractures are more likely to have arterial bleeding
  - Anterior pelvic fractures are more likely to have venous bleeding
- Rectal tears associated with perineal lacerations and associated pelvic fractures (making those open pelvic fractures) may require diverting colostomy

Duodenal Injuries

- Most commonly injured area of duodenum is second portion
- Another common site is at Ligament of Treitz (LOT) where duodenum is tethered.
- Most injuries can be treated with debridement and primary closure alone so long as circumference of bowel after repair is 50% of normal or more
- Resection and end to end closure is often possible with all portions of duodenum except second portion (unfortunately)
- Approximately 25% of patients with significant duodenal injury will die owing to associated injuries & shock
- Post-op fistulae are major source of post-op issues
- Intra-op hematoma >2cm near duodenum needs to be opened for both blunt and penetrating trauma
- Hematoma near duodenum ("paraduodenal") see on CT workup (stable patient) with no obvious duodenal luminal injury
  - Can present with proximal bowel obstruction
  - Do NOT operate or open these
  - Treatment is TPN and NGT. Corrects more than 90% in 2-3 weeks.
  - Being pushed to operate on one? In general, do NOT. Wait longer. NB: two to three WEEKS.
- During laparotomy, if you suspect injury of biliary tree, duodenal, or pancreas injury then medialize duodenum ("Kocher maneuver") and open lesser sac. If you see any evidence of injury (succus, bile, etc.) generally try to formally inspect entire duodenum
- In general with duodenal injuries, try to get primary repair or anastomosis. Remember pyloric exclusion (including gastrojejunostomy) to allow healing. Place feeding tube distal to anastomosis. Place drains liberally around injury.
- Trauma Whipple is rarely if ever indicated

Small bowel injury

- Difficult to diagnose early if isolated and in the setting of blunt trauma
- CT may show free intra-abdominal fluid with NO solid organ injury (if you see that suspect small bowel injury)
- CT may show free intra-abdominal fluid with a solid organ (eg injured spleen) and this may distract from small bowel injury diagnose
- May also see bowel thickening or hematoma at mesentery
- Usually does NOT present with free air seen on xrays done in trauma bay
- Transversely repair lacerations to help avoid stricture
- Resect portion of bowel if injury > 50% bowel circumference or if bowel would be narrow (less than approx. 1/3 diameter of lumen initial size)
- If multiple lacerations close together resect that segment
- Open mesenteric hematomas if larger than 2cm or expanding

Colon injuries

- Right and transverse colon injuries may be repaired primarily
- If unable to repair primarily owing to > 50% circumference injured or associated devascularization, resection and anastomosis
  Diversion not necessary for transverse and right colon injuries
- Primary repair for all LEFT & sigmoid colon injures if less than 50% circumference injured and not associated with devascularization
- If left colectomy or sigmoid colectomy performed because > 50% circumference is injured or devascularization present, create ileostomy in situations where
  - Prolonged time (greater than 6 hours) has passed since initial injury
  - Patient has significant associated disease (eg comorbidities requiring steroid dosing)
  - Substantial transfusions given. Typically greater than 6 units PRBCs.
- In situations where patient is hypotensive / in shock and damage control is being performed, no need to anastamose at index (initial) case. Resect and leave ends in patient for later choice regarding ostomy creation or anastomosis.
- Hematomas near colon are opened whether blunt or penetrating trauma situation.

Rectal injuries

- Presacral drainage and rectal washout are no longer recommended
- Management depends on whether intraperitoneal or extraperitoneal injury
  - Intraperitoneal rectal injury
    - Primary repair without diversion if no significant devascularization and less than 50% circumference
    - If > 50% circumference and / or significant devascularization, low anterior resection with proximal diversion
  - Extraperitoneal rectal injury
    - Proximal 1/3 of rectum: primary repair via laparotomy and proximal diversion
    - Middle 1/3: often inaccessible from beneath and above. May attempt repair but typically create end colostomy only and reverse in approx. 2 months
    - Low: repair primarily via transanal approach ("from beneath") if extensive damage, unable to repair / find lesion: place end colostomy proximally

Liver injuries

- Pringle maneuver issues discussed in hepatobiliary section
- It's rare to need to perform a lobectomy in trauma cases, and some guidelines recommend AGAINST releasing hepatic ligaments and performing lobectomy. So standard ABSITE answer is no lobectomy for trauma...BUT as an FYI some institutions do perform lobectomy in select cases with good outcomes.
- Able to ligate common hepatic artery, because proper hepatic artery will fill via retrograde GastroDuodenal Artery (GDA) flow.
- Atriocaval shunts are performed for retrohepatic IVC injury. May use chest tube or ET tube for actual shunt. Remember IVC control is straightforward in chest and also peri-renal. Can get control at those places and pass shunt.
- Although subcapsular hematomas are to be left alone, portal triad hematomas must be explored. Get control above and below hematoma first with Rummel tourniquets or something similar.
- Common bile duct injury (just FYI I've seen this twice in my career so far)
    - Repair over stent (I've used t tube previously) if < 50%. Remember a pediatric feeding tube (trimmed) is often used as a biliary stent in adults
    - Classic review book recommendation is choledochojejunostomy for injuries greater than 50% circumference. Unfortunately patients with this uncommon injury will not tolerate technically more complex repairs like a "choledocho-j" at index case (first case) in trauma situation. Therefore may need to perform damage control and reconstruct at later case. Unfortunately abdominal contents may be more swollen at takeback for further repair. But of course patient will be alive to get there...
    - Because approximately ten percent of biliary anastomoses leak, if you do perform one, drain area liberally.

- Portal vein injuries must be repaired if at all possible.
    - Sometimes this requires transection of the pancreas to get to the underlying portion if the portal vein in that area.
    - Ligation of the portal vein carries significant risks for mortality. (Approximately 50% mortality.)
- In general, leave drains when there's a liver parenchymal injury
- Hypotensive trauma patients with positive FAST need OR in general as you know.
    - If blunt liver injury is noted and controlled, remember that post operatively (despite appearance of control in OR) patients often require angioembolization.
      Some centers do this angioembolization routinely post op if at all possible based on patient condition.
- In stable patients, non-op management of liver injuries from blunt trauma is the routine plan
    - If patient becomes unstable, resuscitate and go to OR
    - If patient transient responder / requires > 4U PRBCs, angioembolization may be attempted
    - If blush on CT or pseudoaneurysm (in stable patient / transient responder) also may attempt angioembolization.
- Old rule is days of bedrest for blunt liver injuries is grade of injury plus one day. (So a grade 2 injury would be 3 days.) Typically non-operative management involves 5 days bedrest per review book / ABSITE answer.
- Remember hemobilia. (See hepatobiliary chapter.)
- As with splenic injury, grade of injury correlates with risk of failure for non-operative management. It does NOT tell you whether you have to operate on patient—only the risk of failure of non-op management.

Pancreatic injuries

- Contusion: do not open if overlying peritoneum intact when viewed in OR. Place drains overlying
- Most (approximately 80%) of pancreatic injuries are treated with drain placement alone
- Be sure to identify whether pancreatic duct is injured
- CT scans performed initially are often not good at identifying pancreatic injury so maintain suspicion with any question of pancreatic injury on CT
- ERCP often used to find duct injuries and sometimes may treat with stent placement
- Most injuries (80%) are from penetrating trauma
- Distal duct injuries: treat with distal pancreatectomy
- Pancreatic head injuries: drain initially. ERCP with stent later or Whipple later.
- Can take up to approximately 80% of gland before patient becomes diabetic but this is just a rule of thumb
- Older take on this was that you can resect to as far proximal as SMA without patient becoming diabetic (again, rule of thumb)
- Hematomas at the pancreas must be opened whether from penetrating or blunt trauma

Abdominal compartment syndrome (ACS)

- Risk factors include significant fluid resuscitation, abdominal surgery, and trauma
- Bladder pressure > 25-30 suggests ACS
- IVC compression is ultimately what causes decreased venous return and decreased cardiac output
- Diaphragms compressed and moved upward, ventilation difficult, peak airway pressures elevated
- Poor renal perfusion and decreased UOP
- Treatment is decompressive laparotomy, or, if abdomen already open, removal of dressing and new dressing application

Vascular injuries

- Compartment syndrome
    - 5P's are LATE findings. For example loss of pulse does not occur until compartment pressure > systolic blood pressure...BUT compartment syndrome occurs at MUCH lower blood pressures because blood pressure at capillaries in compartments is only approximately 30. So compartment pressures of approximately 30 are usually enough to overcome blood pressures in capillaries and give compartment syndrome. So do NOT wait on the 5Ps.
    - Pain with passive motion may indicate compartment syndrome.
    - Any injury orthopedic injury where blood flow is disrupted for 4-6 hours may give compartment syndrome. Typical examples are humeral fractures (supercondylar), crush injuries of lower extremities, and tibial plateau fractures.
    - So anytime there has been compromised blood flow for 4-6 hours, consider fasciotomy early without waiting for signs to develop later.
- In general, vascular repair first and then orthopedic repair for patient with combined injuries. Shunt first THEN ortho.
- If diminished pulse or signs of distal ischemia beneath level of fracture, reduce fracture first then reassess pulse / ABIs.
- Hard signs of vascular injury (aka Major signs). Go to OR for these
    - Active hemorrhage
    - Pulsatile hematoma
    - No pulse
    - Expanding hematoma
    - Ischemia distal to injury
    - Bruit or thrill at level of injury

- Soft signs (aka Minor signs) of vascular injury. Typically get angio or CTA depending on institution
  - Report of bleeding from site prior to arrival
  - Hematoma, but non-pulsatile
  - Low ABI (less than 0.9)
  - Diminished pulses on one side compared to the other
- GSWs anywhere near popliteal artery need at least high resolution CTA or angiogram even if a palpable pulse is present at dorsalis pedis ipsilateral to injury. This is the exception to a general rule that if there is a pulse present at the foot then there's no need for arterial imaging (even though it typically performed anyway at some institutions). This is because the kinetic energy involved is known to create popliteal intimal flaps which may later cause occlusion or emboli.
- IVC injuries
  - Repair back wall of IVC via venotomy in anterior wall of cava. May need to open front wall to repair suspected injury to back wall.
  - Classic to control IVC proximal and distal to injury with sponge sticks rather than clamps typically
  - Repair IVC if will have patent lumen > or equal to 50% original lumen. If not use patch (saphenous) repair typically if patient condition allows.

Orthopedic injuries

- Avascular necrosis high risk situations include femoral neck fractures with hip dislocations
- Femur fractures may result in 2L of blood loss or more per side
- Fat embolus rate is significantly increased with 2 femur fractures to a surprisingly high approximately 20%
  Fat emboli from long bone fractures present with petechiae, hypoxia, and confusion/agitation. Can try sudan urine stain for fat. Signs of emboli may be visible on eye exam.
- Posterior knee dislocations require formal angiogram (some newer studies claim CTA is adequate given resolution improvements, but standard answer is still arteriogram) unless pulse is absent distal to injury (in which case go to OR)
- In general if pulse absent distal to injury, reduce fracture first.
- If does not return, go to OR. If present but weak, perform CTA.
- Important fractures and associated injuries:
  - Proximal humeral fracture => axillary nerve
  - Should dislocation (anterior and posterior) => axillary nerve
  - Distal humerus fracture => brachial artery
  - Elbow dislocation => brachial artery
  - Distal radial fracture => median nerve
  - Anterior hip dislocation => femoral artery
  - Posterior hip dislocation => sciatic nerve
  - Distal femur fracture => popliteal artery
  - Posterior knee dislocation => popliteal artery
  - Fibula neck fracture => peroneal nerve

Renal injuries

- Remember L renal vein may be ligated near IVC because of gonadal and adrenal collaterals. R renal vein may not and obviously lacks these collaterals.
- Vein, artery, pelvis (renal pelvis) reminds you of structures at renal hilum from anterior to posterior.
- Hematuria seen in trauma bay is the classic sign of renal injury, but other injuries along GU tract may cause this too.
- Greater than 90% of renal injuries are treated without surgical intervention
- Urine extravasation does not guarantee that surgical intervention is necessary; however, after acute injury phase urine extravasation that does not resolve and major collecting system injury ARE indications for intervention
- Intra-operatively, drain area especially any question of collecting system injury
- Remember that IV methylene blue may be used to check for collecting system leak while in the OR
- During ex lap for blunt trauma, hematoma at kidney should NOT be opened unless preop imaging (if you were able to get this) shows severe urine extravasation or non-function of kidney
- During ex lap for penetrating trauma, open hematoma at kidney UNLESS preop imaging demonstrates NO significant urine extravasation and kidney function OK.
- Flank trauma in stable patient with imaging that demonstrates no kidney function: go to angiography

Bladder injury

- Suspect when pelvic fracture present because more than 90% are associated with pelvic fractures
- Hematuria is often another clue
- Blood at penile meatus may be urethral injury or bladder injury
- Cystogram will make diagnosis
- If intraperitoneal, repair with resorbable suture at mucosal layer (PDS or vicryl commonly used) and then two more layers if possible. (Sometimes can only get two layers.) Classic is three layer repair. Remember to look for ureteral orificies and don't close over with repair. Leave foley in place after repair. Intraperitoneal rupture is more common in kids.
- If extraperitoneal, leave foley catheter in place. (1-2 weeks.)

Ureter Injury

- Leave drains if concerned about injured ureter(s) or after repairing ureters
- Large segment of ureter missing (over 2 cm)
    - Distal third injured
      mobilize ureter and reimplant in bladder. May need bladder hitch (psoas hitch) to bring bladder up to ureter a bit for anastomosis

    - Not distal third
        - Tie off both ends of ureter
        - Perc nephrostomy placement
        - Later on, may reconstruct with trans ureteroureterostomy (uses contralateral ureter) or ileal interposition
- Small segment missing
    - Distal third injured
      Reimplant into bladder as above. Again may need psoas hitch.

    - Not distal third
        - Mobilize ends and perform anastomosis over a stent
        - Typically PDS is suture used
        - Ends of ureter are beveled if at all possible to avoid stricture.
- IVP with one shot does not adequately eval ureters for injury
- Remember Methylene blue or indigo carmine (IV) checks for leaks

Trauma to urethra & miscellaneous GU

- Males much more common given urethral length, etc.
- Pelvic fractures (particularly open book), blood at meatus, prostate gland not palpable or "free floating", hematuria...all signs of possible urethral injury
- Do NOT place a foley if injury suspected
- Perform RUG (Retrograde UrethroGram)
- Portion of urethra most at risk for injury is membranous portion
- Partial tears that are small may be treated with catheter bridging repair and delayed definitive repair (months later)
- Suprapubic cystostomy is performed if significant tear. Definitive repair is performed MONTHS later owing to high rate of stricture and possible impotence with immediate / early repair.
- Penile fracture from sex or other trauma: need to repair Buck's fascia and tunica
- If testicular trauma, do ultrasound to check flow and tunica albuginea. Repair tunica if needed.

Pediatric Trauma

- < 1 YOA has typical vitals of HR > 160, SBP > 80, RR < 40
- 1 to 5 YOA typical vitals are HR > 140, SBP > 90, RR < 30
- Greater 10 YOA typical vitals are HR > 120, SBP > 100, RR < 20
- remember pediatric patients will compensate for blood loss very effectively and for a long time until they suddenly can't anymore. They "fall off a cliff" late when they finally can't compensate anymore. Maintain high index of suspicion for shock and blood loss.
- Pediatric patients have an increased risk of both head injury and hypothermia

Pregnant patients and trauma

- 33% of total intravascular volume may be lost by pregnant patients prior to them demonstrating physical signs
- Resuscitation and treatment is primarily directed toward the mother first. "Mother first" or "save the mother at all costs".
- To help estimate how far along pregnancy is, remember that fundus of uterus is at umbilicus at 20 weeks. So 20 weeks gestation is approximately 20cm height and at umbilicus.
- in first trimester, avoid CT if possible. Remember ultrasound and MRI may be useful for imaging the area too.
- Vaginal discharge including blood or amnion is concerning.
- C-section during trauma laparotomy if
  - Severe intra-uterine trauma
  - Severe injuries / shock in mother and pregnancy near term (greater than 34 wks)
  - Continued pregnancy is threat to mother owing to DIC or bleeding
  - Unable to expose injured vessels in pelvis owing to uterus present

Miscellaneous facts about pulmonary function that often come up in trauma / ICU patients:

- Pulmonary compliance = change in Volume for a given change in Pressure (want high compliance)
  Compliance decreased in ARDS, pulmonary edema (takes greater pressure to get same volume)
- Aging reduces FEV1 and FVC
- Initial Rx for air embolus is place pt in Tendelenburg with L side down. Can then attempt air aspiration via central line placed to depth of right atrium
- PEEP (Positive End Expiratory Pressure) increases functional residual capacity (FRC), increased compliance. Also keeps alveoli open. Penumothorax unusual unless very high
- FRC is volume in lungs after normal exhalation
- Inspiratory capacity: air breathed in from FRC
- Vital capacity: greatest volume that can be exhaled

Miscellaneous

- Endothelial derived relaxing factor, aka nitric oxide (NO), is produced from arginine in endothelial cells. Increased in sepsis. Produces vasodilatation. NO is released in response to serial compression device (SCD) function. This is why SCDs placed on the upper extremities (not just the lower extremities) give some risk reduction for DVT.
- Hydroflouric acid burns treated with topical calcium
- Carbon monoxide falsely elevates the O2 sat. Hemoglobin dissociation curve is left shifted. Cherry red lips may be seen in trauma bay. 100% oxygen administration reduces half life of CO to 1 hour from 5 hours.
- Silvadene: neutropenia risk. Activity against Candida is good. Eschar penetration is poor.
- Sulfamylon: **painful**; acidosis is due to carbonic anhydrase inhibition (Less bicarb going to H2O + CO2 so therefore acidotic.)
- Silver Nitrate: hyponatremia & hypochloremia due to NaCl loss
- electrical burns can give rhabdo, compartment syndrome, cataracts, hollow viscus perforation, solid organ injuries...immediate death may result from vfib
- Most common infection in burn patients is *pneumonia*
- Burn patients have an initial decrease in cardiac output, then an increase later. (Hyperdynamic.)
- Marjolin's ulcer is squamous cell cancer that develops in a chronic wound

Thyroid

From endoderm. 3rd week of gestation, thyroid descends from foramen cecum to just above cricoid. From 1st and 2nd pharyngeal arches not pouches.

Ultimobrachial bodies (from neurectoderm at 4th brachial pouch) give rise to C cells that produce calcitonin. Calcitonin antagonizes PTH. Calcitonin shifts calcium into bones: "Calcitonin puts the bone in".

Arterial supply from the inferior thyroid artery (from the thyrocervical trunk) & superior thyroid artery (first branch of external carotid)

Drainage is via the superior, middle, and inferior thyroid veins. Inferior drains into the innominate. Superior and middle drain into the internal jugular.

Recurrent Laryngeal Nerves (RLNs)

- RLNs from the vagus innervate all intrinsic laryngeal muscles except cricothyroid.
- Ligament of Berry is suspensory ligament located posteriorly near RLN.
- Left RLN branch loops around the aorta at ligamentum arteriosum & ultimately sits in tracheoesophageal groove
- Right RLN loops around the right subclavian artery.
- RLNs are associated with inferior thyroid arteries. So don't ligate the inferior thyroid arteries unless you're sure you are NOT ligating RLN along with them.
- In 1-2% of people, RLN is not recurrent. More common to be non-recurrent on right side.
- Injury gives hoarseness. Bilateral injury may cause airway obstruction and need for tracheostomy.
- Superior laryngeal nerve arises from vagus and gives internal and external branches. This is the most commonly injured nerve with thyroidectomy. Injury gives inability to project voice and early voice fatigue so that's a potential issue for singers.
- Internal branch provides sensation to the larynx
- External branch gives motor function to cricothyroid muscle.

T4 is the major hormone produced in the thyroid. 80–85% production. T3 is made in thyroid and also via peripheral conversion of T4. T3 is more active and has a shorter half-life.

A TSH and Free T4 level will tell you whether patient is hypo or hyperthyroid.

Thyroid Releasing Factor (TRF) from hypothalamus acts on anterior pituitary to cause release of thyroid stimulating hormone (TSH)

TSH acts on thyroid to cause release of T4 and T3.

A thyroid mass is evaluated by an FNA. If can't palpate or near vascular structures, US guided biopsy

Thyroid storm

- Symptoms include increased HR, fever, high output cardiac failure (most frequent cause of death), numbness
- Typically seen in patient with unrecognized Graves' disease who undergoes a surgical procedure.
- Wolff-Chaikoff effect: patient given Lugol's solution (high does iodine) which leads to inhibition of TSH action on thyroid and coupling of iodine, therefore less T4 and T3
- Treatment = beta blockers, steroids, iodine and propylthiouracil (PTU)
- Indications for thyroidectomy in hyperthyroidism include tracheal compression, thyrotoxicosis, and cosmesis
- In pregnancy, do NOT give radioiodine. PTU only.

Hyperthyroidism

- Increased free T4, low TSH
- Grave's disease is most common cause
- Especially in women 20-40
- HLA B8 and DR3 are associated with Grave's
- Moist skin, afib, tachycardia, goiter, pretibial myxedema, ophthalmic issues
- In addition to free T4 elevation and decreased TSH, will see thyroid receptor autoantibodies
- Initial therapy is medical. If fails medical treatment, patient has large goiter, or is pregnant, surgical intervention is indicated.

Thyroiditis

- In general, salicylates are given to different types of thyroiditis for symptomatic relief.
- Acute suppurative is due to bacterial infection. May be from bacterial URI (staph/strep). WBC elevation. Treatment is antibiotics and I&D of abscesses.
- Subacute
    - DeQuervain's is due to viral infection. May be preceded by viral URI, ASA, NSAIDS, steroids are treatment options and typically this resolves in 4-6 months. Typical changes of hyperthyroidism on labs: increased free T4 and TSH low. However **ESR (sed rate) is elevated**.
    - Postpartum thyoiditis is an autoimmune condition. Occurs in postpartum period. Treat symptoms. Looks like DeQuervain's except **ESR is normal**.
- Chronic
    - Hashimoto's is an autoimmune condition. **Painless** inflammation of gland. Initially hyperthyroidism (with labs consistent) then later hypothyroidism. **Anti-thyroid antibody positive, antithyroperoxidase antibody positive.** May treat hypothyroid phase with thyroid hormone replacement. Thyroid cancer can develop in a patient with Hashimoto's thyroiditis, so maintain a high index of suspicion for conditions like thyroid lymphoma / nodules.
    - Riedel's struma is painless "woody" inflammation of gland. Lymphocyte infiltrate of gland seen. Resect thyroid stromal tissue (isthmectomy or tracheostomy) to relieve compressive symptoms. Treat with thyroxine and steroids.

Hypothyroidism

- Common causes include thyroid resection, I-131 ablation, thyroiditis, medications (eg lithium and amiodarone)
- Symptoms include weight gain, constipation, thinning hair, cold intolerance, pretibial myxedema
- Cretinism is congenital hypothyroidism
- Treat with levothyroxine
- Myxedema coma is associated with a high mortality rate. Secure airway, achieve normothermia, and treat with IV T4 (thyroxine)
- 5H's of myxedema coma: hypotension, hypothermia, hypoventilation, hyponatremia, hypoglycemia

Thyroid cancer

- most frequent endocrine malignancy (in US)
- 5-10% chance of malignancy if follicular cells seen on FNA
- follicular adenoma: still need lobectomy to prove it's benign adenoma
- cold nodules, male patient, age > 50 all worrisome for cancer

- Papillary cancer
    - 80% of cancers
    - women 20-40 YOA
    - associated with exposure to radiation
    - spreads via lymphatics
    - MAJORITY of these present with metastasis, but that is NOT prognostic of outcome
    - Remember "lateral ectopic thyroid" or node biopsy that says normal thyroid tissue is actually metastatic papillary cancer.
    - SO...if you biopsy a lymph node in the neck and pathology comes back "ectopic thyroid tissue" or "benign thyroid tissue" it's NOT benign thyroid tissue...it's papillary thyroid cancer.
    - Psammoma bodies and orphan annie cells seen on pathology
    - If < 1cm, lobectomy and isthmusectomy is standard. Some argue though that total thyroidectomy is justified because papillary cancer is multicentric and diffuse
    - If > 1cm, high risk, or bilateral do total thyroidectomy
    - If + central node at neck, do central node dissection
    - If lateral node positive at neck, do modified radical neck dissection.
    - Give iodine 131 postop if lesion > 1.5cm (unless pregnant)
    - Follow thyroglobulin levels post op because will help indicate tumor reurrence
    - Approximately 95% five year survival. In the 5% who do die, death is from local disease.
    - AMES and TNM system may be used to determine mortality risk
    - Age is the biggest prognostic factor for thyroid cancer.

- Follicular cancer
  - Most common type in women > 50 YOA
  - Represents about 10% of thyroid cancer cases
  - Hurthle cell variant is more likely to be both multifocal and bilateral
  - Hurthle cells are eonsinophilic cells that increase the rate of lymphatic spread
  - However, in general, follicular CA demonstrates hematogenous spread.
  - FNA demonstrates microfollicles.
  - Treatment is lobetomy or total thyroidectomy
  - If cancer persists or recurs after lobectomy, perform completion thyroidectomy and treat with postop iodine 131. Follow thyroglobulin levels.
  - Five year survival approximately 70% except Hurthle cell does give increased mortality rate.
- Post op iodine 131 yes or no?
  - Consider I 131 6 weeks after surgery, when TSH is at maximum. This allows maximal response.
  - Tumor > 1cm
  - Disease outside of thyroid
  - Need total thyroidectomy for iodine 131 to be effective
- Choice of surgical procedure for Papillary and Follicular
  - Lobectomy if does not meet total thyroidectomy indications beneath
  - Total thyroidectomy if
    - Lesion > 1cm
    - Disease outside of thyroid
    - Multi-focal or bilateral disease
    - Previous xray therapy to neck

- Anaplastic cancer
    - Most common type in women over 65 YOA, but represents approx. 3% of cancers overall.
    - Often shows up with metastatic disease at time of diagnosis. Poorly differentiated or undifferentiated.
    - Any resection is for improvement of airway issues only
    - TWO year survival is approximately 10%. Most commonly patients only survive approximately 4 months.
- Medullary
    - Incidence in men vs. women the same. 5% of cases.
    - ¼ of patients have MEN-2 (see bilateral disease more often and multicentric disease more often). RET mutation causes MEN.
    - increased calcitonin owing to hyperplastic C cells. This cancer arises from C cells.
    - increased CEA
    - see amyloid on biopsy that gives "apple green birefringence"? Then that's medullary carcinoma of the thyroid and may be associated with MEN. Remember to look for the adrenal lesion that may be associated and reset that first after routine preparations.
    - Perform total thyroidectomy and central node dissection
    - NO iodine 131 for medullary CA
    - If nodes positive, approximately 40% survival at ten years. If nodes negative, approximately 80%.
- Lymphoma
    - 1% of thyroid CA cases. More common in women
    - seen with Hashimoto's thyroiditis.
    - Non-Hodgkin's type
    - May need airway intervention if expands quickly
    - 50% five year survival
    - drops to 35% if extrathyroidal disease is present

MEN 2

- Both MEN 2A and MEN 2B are due to autosomal dominant mutation in RET on chromosome 10.
- Both MEN 2A and MEN 2B include medullary carcinoma of the thyroid and pheochromocytoma.
- When you find a family with MEN 2 remember that the children will inherit the disease from biologic parents. So if you find yourself discovering a medullary carcinoma of the thyroid in an adult, recall that 25% are MEN 2 related, test chromosome 10 and find RET mutation...remember that any biologic children will have the gene as well. So follow the recommendations beneath regarding thyroidectomy for them.
- MEN 2A (Sipple syndrome)
    - In addition to above, includes hyperparathyroidism
    - Test for RET
    - Prophylactic thyroidectomy by 5 years of age
- MEN 2B
    - As above with marfanoid body habitus and mucosal neuromas, but NO hyperparathyroidism.
    - Also, prophylactic thyroidectomy should be performed in infancy.

Parathyroid

Superior glands are from 4th brachial pouch

Inferior glands (and thymus) from 3rd brachial pouch

90% of patients have all 4 parathyroid glands

- Superior glands are usually located posterolaterally to RLN
- Classic ectopic gland locations
    - Superior glands missing? Look in
        - Tracheoesophageal groove
        - Tracheal bifurcation
        - Retroesophageal space
        - Retropharyngeal space
        - Carotid sheath
    - Inferior glands missing? Look in
        - Intrathyroidal position
        - Carotid sheath

Composed of Chief cells (secrete PTH) and oxyphil cells

Blood supply is from inferior thyroid artery, which runs in close association with RLNs

Parathyroid hormone causes bone resorption by activating osteoclasts, increased vitamin D activation at kidney via 1 alpha hydroxylase, increased inorganic phosphate excretion, increased calcium resorption by kidneys.

Increased Ca^{++} causes DECREASED PTH release

Serum magnesium needs to be calcium before repleting Ca^{++}. That's because magnesium affects calcium regulation and low magnesium inhibits PTH. This is why Chvostek's sign and other signs of hypocalcemia (Trousseau's sign, tetany) may also be seen with low magnesium.

Calcitonin from C cells of thyroid antagonizes PTH effects

"Moans, stones, groans [bone pain] & psychiatric overtones" are the signs of hypercalcemia associated with hyperparathyroidism.

Hypercalcemic crisis is treated with "forced diuresis": saline and Lasix. May see short QT and absent ST segment. Cortisone and mithramycin may be used.

Parathyroid cancer

- Rare
- Ca++ levels typically greater than 14. Higher than what's usually seen with hyperparathyroidism.
- Resect en bloc any involved structures, including parathyroid, thyroid, and anything else involved.
- May look benign on histology so this is a difficult diagnosis
- 50-75% five year survival.

Familial hypocalciuric hypercalcemia: does NOT require parathyroidectomy or surgical treatment of any kind

See increased serum calcium and DECREASED urine calcium (in hyperparaythyroidism, see increased serum calcium and INCREASED urine calcium)

MEN 1 (Wermer's)

- Menin gene mutation on chromosome 11
- Autosomal dominant
- Prolactinoma (pituitary tumor)
- Four gland hyperplasia (hyperparathyroidism)
- Neuroendocrine / pancreatic tumor
  Most common gastrinoma (in gastrinoma triangle)

Types of hyperparathyroidism

- Primary
    - Single adenoma causes 85% of cases
    - 4 gland hyperplasia & carcinoma can cause
    - see increased PTH
    - increased serum calcium and increased urine calcium
    - low serum phosphate
    - perform parathyroidectomy for issues related to hypercalcemia
    - for adenoma, resect adenoma
    - for hyperplasia, remove 3 and ½ glands and autotransplant (putting transplant in forearm allows blood pressure cuff to be inflated proximally to check whether transplant is working. Inflating cuff should decrease serum PTH if transplant working.)
- Secondary
    - Chronic renal failure
    - Increased PTH
    - Normal or even DECREASED serum calcium
    - Increased serum phosphate
    - Parathyroidectomy, phosphate binders, remember that calciphylaxis may occur
- Tertiary
    - Continued autonomous PTH release after renal transplant
    - Increased PTH and serum calcium
    - Decreased serum phosphate
    - Parathyroidectomy if continues 1 year after transplant

Adrenal

Adrenal cortex is mesoderm

Adrenal medulla is from neural crest ectoderm

Extra-adrenal locations for neural crest ectoderm include retroperitoneal rests and Organ of Zuckerkandl at aortic bifrucation

Has cortex (Greek for "bark" because it's on the outside like bark of a tree) and medulla

Cortex is divided into

- Zona glomerulosa
    - Makes mineralocorticoids (aldosterone)
    - Conn's syndrome is hyperaldosteronism leading to hypertension and hypokalemia
        - weakness, polydipsia and polyuria are seen
        - Salt load suppression test: salt load patient and urine aldosterone stays high
        - Aldosterone to renin ratio: > 20:1
        - Low serum K+, high serum Na+, metabolic alkalosis
        - Primary Conn's has low renin and adenoma is cause of 85% of cases of primary Conn's
        - Secondary Conn's has elevated renin. Secondary is more common than primary, seen with CHF, renal artery stenosis, aldosteronoma
    - Aldosteronoma
        - Aldosterone is released when stimulation occurs from renin-angiotensin-aldosterone system and decreased blood volume. Gives increased Na+ resorption at nephron (distal portion). H+ and K+ increased secretion. (all are normal physiology)
            - Most commonly single adenoma (70%), may be bilateral hyperplasia (30%) HTN, hypokalemia, nonanion gap metabolic acidosis
            - HTN, hypokalemia, nonanion gap metabolic acidosis are seen
            - Serum aldosterone and serum aldosterone to renin ratio elevated
            - If aldosterone:renin elevated and no mass, or bilateral adrenal lesions are present, consider adrenal vein sampling. If sampling localizes, remove ipsilateral adrenal. If no localization, start spironolactone.
        - Most commonly single adenoma (70%), may be bilateral hyperplasia (30%) HTN, hypokalemia, nonanion gap metabolic acidosis
        - HTN, hypokalemia, nonanion gap metabolic acidosis
        - Serum aldosterone and serum aldosterone to renin ratio elevated
        - If aldosterone:renin elevated and no mass, or bilateral adrenal lesions are present, consider adrenal vein sampling. If sampling localizes, remove ipsilateral adrenal. If no localization, start spironolactone.

- Zona fasciculata
  - Glucocorticoids (cortisol)
    - Pregenolone converted to cortisol when stimulation from ACTH occurs via enzymatic conversions involving 3 hydroxylases: 21, 11 beta, and 17 alpha.
    - Addison's disease (low cortisol) most common cause is withdraw of exogenous steroids
      - Most common PRIMARY cause is autoimmune disease
      - May also be seen with decreased aldosterone
      - Cosyntropin stim test to diagnose (give ACTH and measure serum cortisol)
    - Acute adrenal insufficiency: refractory hypotension (despite pressors and fluids) give dexamethasone (will NOT interfere with cosyntropin stim test) More on adrenal insufficiency later in section.
      Waterhouse-Friedrichson is adrenal insufficiency owing to adrenal hemorrhage. May be seen with sepsis.

    - Cushing's syndrome (hypercortisolism) most commonly due to exogenous steroid dosing
      - Measure 24 hour urine cortisol and ACTH
      - If ACTH low and cortisol high patient has cortisol secreting lesion
      - If ACTH and cortisol are high, patient has pituitary adenoma or an ectopic source of ACTH
        So, give high dose dexamethasone suppression test. If urine cortisol decreases, patient has pituitary lesion. If not, has ectopic ACTH production (eg small cell lung CA).

- Zona reticularis
  - Sex steroids (dihydroepiandrosterone)
    - Results in eventual production of testosterone
    - From DHEA or 17 alpha hydroxyprogesterone

Medulla is composed of chromaffin cells that make norepinephrine and epinephrine

- These catecholamines are produced from tyrosine. Pathway is tyrosine to L DOPA to dopamine to norepinephrine then finally epinephrine.
- Tyrosine to L DOPA is rate limiting step (tyrosine hydrolase)
- PNMT converts norepi to epi
  PNMT (phenylethanolamine N methyltransferase) enzyme is ONLY found in adrenal medulla
- Byproducts including vanillylmandelic acid (VMA) and homovanillic acid are made
  MAO (monoamine oxidase) enzyme converts breaks down catecholamines to produce these

Supplied by middle adrenal artery (from aorta), superior adrenal artery (from phrenic), and inferior adrenal artery (from renal artery)

Most blood that eventually cortex enters passes through medulla first

Usually one adrenal vein on each side: on R drains to IVC, on L drains to renal vein

"Incidentaloma" at adrenal

- adrenal lesion found when patient worked up for other things, eg pan-CT scan for trauma patient
- lesions may be functional or non-functional and benign or malignant
- malignancy risk by size
  - less than 4 cm has approx. 2% risk of cancer
  - 4-6 cm has approximately 6% risk of cancer
  - greater than 6 cm has 25% risk of cancer
- 5% are metastastatic lesions
- rule out functional mass first with urine metanephrines, VMA, catecholamines, urinary hydroxycorticosteroids, serum potassium levels, and plasma renin and aldosterone levels
- foreboding CT scan signs include lesion > 4-6 cm, enlarging lesion over time, non-homogenous appearance
- CXR, mammogram, and colonoscopy may be performed to check for primary tumor if metastasis suspected
- metastases to adrenals: lung CA most common, breast, melanoma, renal cell CA
- biopsy lesions (especially if cancer history) AFTER ruling out functional lesion
- non-functional lesions > 4-6 cm should be removed owing to cancer risk. So rather than needle biopsy, remove lesion. Use of laparoscopic approach has been decreasing the size criteria felt to be appropriate for resection.
- If you decide to follow an incidental adrenal lesion over time rather than resect, repeat imaging every three months for first year followed by yearly thereafter.

Congenital Adrenal Hyperplasia

- Most commonly due to lack of 21 hydroxylase
- Decreased aldosterone and decreased cortisol
- Virilization seen as well as hypotension
- Decreased Na+, increased K+
- Increased 17 alpha progesterone
- Increased androstenedione
- Increased testosterone

Adrenal insufficiency

- Seen in up to 30% of critically ill ICU patients
- Primary is due to failure of gland owing to stress, atrophy, hemorrhage (again Waterhouse-Friedrichsen syndrome), etc.
- Symptoms range from subtle (hyperpigmentation, weight loss, hyperpigmentation, abdominal pain) to severe (hypotension despite pressors)
- May see decreased Na+, increased K+, nongap metabolic acidosis
- Perform cosyntropin stim test

Pheochromocytoma

- From chromaffin cells
- right sided lesions are more common
- extra-adrenal lesions are more commonly malignant
- Most common location is adrenal gland, but may be seen in Organ of Zuckerkandl
- 10% malignant, 10% bilateral, 10% familial (remember MEN syndromes), 10% seen in children, 10% extra-adrenal
- also associated with von Recklinghausen's (chromosome 17 easily remember because "von Recklinghausen" has 17 letters in it), Sturge-Weber, and tuberous sclerosis
- MIBG scan will identify location if you are unable to see lesion on CT
- 24 hour urine metanephrines is the best test, also send VMA
- lesion does NOT respond to clonidine suppression test
- preop: volume load patient first, give alpha blockade (prazosin, phenoxybenzamine), THEN add beta-blocker if arrhythmias or tachycardia seen. Do NOT add beta blockade before alpha blockade or patient may develop hypertensive crisis with stroke, MI, heart failure
- nipride and neosynephrine as well as anti-arrhythmics should be readily available during surgery
- during adrenalectomy, ligate adrenal vein first to avoid spilling catecholamines during lesion manipulation
- metyrosine inhibits tyrosine hydroxylase causing decreased catecholamine synthesis

Skin and Soft Tissue

Layers

- Epidermis, composed of stratified squamous epithelium, contains
    - Keratinocytes (main cell type)
    - Melanocytes
        - Melanin is transferred to keratinocytes via melanosomes
        - Races all have same "density" of melanocytes…difference is in amount of melanin produced
    - Merkel cells
    - Langerhan's cells
        - From bone marrow
        - MHC class 2 antigen presenting cells
    - Basal membrane
      Anchors dermis to epidermis

    - Dermis, approx. 70% composed of type 1 collagen (which provides tensile strength), contains
        - Dermal appendages
        - Hair follicles (which contain cells that can later differentiate for wound healing)
        - Meissner's corpuscles: sense light touch
        - Pacinian corpuscles: sense pressure

Free flaps and pedicled flaps share most common cause of necrosis: venous thrombosis

Squamous cell cancer

- Occurs in sun exposed areas (eg lower lip & backs of hands)
- Risk factors
  - UV / ionizing radiation exposure is risk factor
  - Presence of actinic keratosis is risk factor
  - Tobacco use
  - Chronic infection (such as HPV infection)
  - Immunosuppression (as in organ transplant patients)
  - Burns (Marjolin's ulcer is a type of squamous cell cancer)
  - Chronic, non-healing wounds
- Red, itchy plaque with central bleeding, ulceration, or pruritis
- Clinical diagnosis usually but may be confirmed with biopsy
- Path on biopsy shows atypical keratinocytes invading the dermis. Keratin pearls also seen.
- Most common cancer seen in solid organ transplant patients (followed by Post-Transplant Lymphoproliferative Disease and then Kaposi's sarcoma)
- Bowen's disease is squamous cell carcinoma in situ
  - Associated with HPV
  - Try to avoid excision if at all possible owing to recurrence (owing to HPV)
  - Treatments include imiquimod, cautery to ablate, topical 5-FU
- Excise lesion with 1cm margin. Perform lymph node excision if palpable node(s)
- Squamous cell cancer more likely to metastasize than basal cell cancer. And prognosis is worse than basal cell cancer.
- 3 year survival for all comers is 85%. Much lower if patients have metastasis

Basal cell cancer

- Most are located on head and neck (80%)
- Most common malignancy in United States, and 4 times more likely than squamous cell cancer (except in transplant population)
- Arises in epidermis and is slow growing
- Pathology demonstrates stromal retraction as well as peripheral palisading of nuclei
- Node disease and metastases are rarely seen
- If nodes are clinically positive, perform regional node dissection
- Most aggressive type is morpheaform type. Makes collagenase.
- Resect with 0.3 to 0.5 cm margins. Chemo and radiation therapy have very limited role confined to inoperable disease, metastasis, or neurovascular invasion

Glomus tumor

- glomus body normally regulates perfusion to distal digit
- glomus tumor is benign tumor on digit that includes blood vessel and nerve structures arising from glomus body
- often subungual position
- typically seen in women aged 30-50 years
- seen as bluish nodule beneath nail
- any symptoms are worse with cold exposure
- usually < 1 cm blanching nodule
- remove with approach via nail bed or approach laterally if at nail margin

Soft tissue and skin syndromes

- Familial Atypical Multiple Mole Melanoma (FAMMM syndrome)
  - Diagnostic criteria
    - One or more first or second degree relatives with melanoma
    - Many moles (typically > 50) with atypical characteristics such as asymmetrical, raised, or different colors)
    - Moles with specific microscopic appearances
    - Increased risk for pancreatic cancer with FAMMM
  - Genetic facts
    - Autosomal dominant inheritance
    - CDKN2A (p16) on chromosome 9
    - CDK4 on chromosome 12
    - Related to how cell cycle continues in G1-S transition
- Tuberous sclerosis
  - Hamartomas seen in lung, brain, kidney
  - Epilepsy & retardation
  - Shagreen patches, ash leaf macules, & adenoma sebaceum all seen
  - Angiomyolipoma associated with this condition
  - Genetics
    - TSC1 on chromosome 9
    - TSC2 on chromosome 16
    - Regulate GTPase activity

- Gardner's syndrome
  - GI polyps (eg ampullary, small intestine, large intestine)
  - Desmoid tumors
  - Sebaceous cysts and osteomas
  - Genetics
    - Related to familial adenomatous polyposis (variant)
    - Adenomatous Polyposis Coli (APC) gene on chromosome 5
    - Autosomal dominant
  - Gene is involved in cytoskeleton and cell adhesion
- Neurofibromatosis type 1
  - Also known as von Recklinghausen's disease
  - Lisch nodules (which are hamartomas at iris)
  - Café au lait spots (which are hyperpigmented macules)
  - Optic gliomas
  - Freckles at non-sun exposed areas such as groin and axillae
  - Increased risk for astrocytomas, pheochromocytomas, and neurofibrosarcomas
  - Genetics
    - NF1 gene (chromosome 17, remember 17 letters in "von Recklinghausen")
    - Autosomal dominant
    - Gene is related to ras pathway
    - More commonly seen than Neurofibromatosis type 2
- Neurofibromatosis type 2
  Bilateral cranial nerve 8 (acoustic nerve) lesions. These are schwannomas
- Intracranial / intraspinal tumors
- Genetics
- NF2 gene on chromosome 22, related to in cytoskeleton creation
- Autosomal dominant

Pyoderma gangrenosum

- Necrotic ulcer with violate / purple colored borders and surrounding erythema
- Associated with ulcerative colitis, regional ileitis, rheumatoid arthritis, leukemia, lymphoma
- Treat with systemic steroids and cyclosporine, sometimes require skin grafts
- Patients may respond to bowel resection if underlying condition is bowel issue

Tranverse Rectus Abdominus Myocutaneous (TRAM) flaps

- share most common cause of necrosis with free flaps: venous thrombosis (pedicled flaps and free flaps both most commonly necrose owing to venous thrombosis)
- complications include hernia, infection, abdominal wall weakness, and flap necrosis
- depend on the superior epigastric vessels
- most important determinant of viability is muscle perforators in periumbilical area.

Presence of melanin is best factor for protecting skin from UV radiation damage. UV radiation causes direct DNA damage and also damages DNA repair mechanisms. UV-B radiation is cause of chronic sun damage.

Melanoma

- Ulcerations, male gender, mucosal or ocular lesion worse prognosis
- Don't shave skin lesions that may be melanoma because shave biopsies won't reveal depth which is required to determine depth and extent of margins for resection
- Diagnostic biopsies
    - Lesion less than 2cm: perform excisional biopsy unless lesion is in a sensitive area. May also use Tru-Cut or core needle biopsy if lesion is in difficult area. Remember the idea is to get depth of lesion and if lesion is melanoma then may return and resect with margins
    - Greater than 2cm: incisional biopsy eg punch biopsy. Remember to include both portion of lesion and margin of normal surrounding tissue as this allows comparison by pathologist. If positive will need to return and resect with margins.
- Types
    - lentigo maligna
      radial growth initially, least aggressive, may present as raised nodule

    - Superficial spreading
      Most common type. Sometimes starts in a nevus.

    - acral lentiginous
      much more aggressive than other types except nodular. May be beneath nails (subungual). Arises on palms / soles of feet.

    - Nodular
      Most aggressive type. Typically has metastasized at time of diagnosis. Vertical growth first. May occur anywhere.

- For all melanoma > 1mm, examine ALL nodal basins that may drain area of lesion (sometime this includes contralateral side), inferior / superior basin), CT chest/abdomen/pelvis, LFTs, and LDH.
- Requires wide local excision with these margins
    - Melanoma in situ, thin lentigo maligna (aka Hutckinson's freckle) in epidermis only: 0.5 cm margins
    - 1cm for lesion < or equal to 1mm depth except as above. Note that 0.1 mm to 1.0 mm depth is T1 lesion.
    - 1-2 cm for lesions 1.1-2 mm (remember sentinel node biopsy too) Note that 1.01 to 2.0 depth is T2 lesion
    - 2 cm for lesions 2-4 mm (sentinel node biopsy too) 2.01-4.0 depth is T3 lesion, etc.
    - 2-3 cm for lesions > 4 mm (sentinel node biopsy too)
    - SLN (sentinel node biopsy) for all lesions > 1mm thickness even if no palpable nodes. If palpable nodes, SLN for all lesions greater than 0.75mm thickness
- Leading cause of skin cancer death (65% of deaths) but represents only approx. 5% of cases
    - Risk factors include
        - congenital nevi, dysplastic nevi, atypical nevi
        - Familial BK mole syndrome
        - Xeroderma pigmentosum
        - Previous XRT
        - Multiple sunburns, history of easy burning
- Most common location in women is on legs, & most common location in men is on back
- Although the most common metastasis TO the small bowel is melanoma, the most common location for distant metastasis is the lungs
- ABCDE for signs of melanoma: A is asymmetry in shape of skin lesion, B is borders that are irregular, C is changing color eg darkening of lesions, D is increasing diameter, and E is Elevation of lesion
- Clark's and Breslow's levels do NOT align with TNM staging and do NOT line up with the recommendations for margins on resection that are listed above. Review them if you have a moment but do not use to decide on margins.
- Rules for TNM staging
    - Presence of metastasis makes patient stage 4 no matter what else with tumor or nodes
    - Presence of ANY number of positive nodes makes stage 3, NO positive nodes means must be stage 1 or 2
    - Stage 1 requires lesion 2.0 mm or less WITHOUT ulceration. (T2a with "a" means no ulceration. "b" means ulceration)

      Example: T2bN1M0 is Stage 3 lesion. T2bN0M0 is stage 2 lesion, not stage 1 because ulceration present. T2aN1M1 is stage 4 lesion because metastasis. T2aN0M0 is stage 1 lesion.

Merkel Cell Carcinoma

- Purple or red painless nodule of head or neck
- Stains with neuron specific enolase (NSE) to confirm diagnosis. May also stain with neurofilament protein.
- May be associated with metachronous or synchronous squamous cell cancer
- Treatment is excision with 3cm margins
- All patients get sentinel node biopsy or node dissection. High rate of nodal involvement owing to early regional and systemic spread.
- 30-40% five year survival
- Neuroendocrine lesion

Keratoses

- Arsenical
  Lesion is more commonly associated with squamous cell cancer

- Seborrheic
  Typically located centrally (trunk) on elderly patient. NOT premalignant.

- Actinic
  Premalignant. Needs removal if suspicious of malignancy at all. Liquid nitrogen or diclofenac may be used as treatments. Occurs in areas that are sun damaged.

Desmoid

- Benign tumor typically seen in 3rd to 4th decade of life
- May present as obstruction
- Biopsy shows spindle cells surrounded by collagen
- Difficult surgical management owing to size and invasion of surrounding structures
- Associated with Gardner's syndrome (subtype of familial adenomatous polyposis)
- Associated with retroperitoneal fibrosis
- May encase bowel making resection difficult
- Sulindac or tamoxifen as chemotherapy if vital structure involved or patient would be left with short gut
- Excise with 2 to 4 cm margins if possible

Rectus sheath hematoma

- Almost never need to operate; however, resuscitate and correct coagulopathy (eg DDAVP in renal failure patients, etc.)
- From injury to collaterals of superior or inferior epigastric or directly to artery
- Fothergill's sign is mass becomes more evident with tensing rectus muscles
- Embolization is an option if needs urgent treatment beyond resuscitation
- Operative intervention is rarely required

Kaposi's sarcoma

- Associated with HIV and AIDS, immunosuppression, chemotherapy, and also herpes virus 8.
- Most frequent AIDS related malignancy
- Purple or red nodule on skin or mucosa
- Biopsy to diagnose
- Primary goal of treatment is to palliate
- Treat underlying condition (eg AIDS)
    - Use HAART therapy
    - Intra-lesion vinblastine and x-ray therapy are other options
    - Interferon alpha may be used for disseminated disease
    - If severe GI bleed, may require surgery despite obvious higher risks given CD4 count and issues with healing
- Resection is reserved for lesions that interfere with vital bodily processes (resection is rare)

Osteosarcoma

- Most common bone malignancy.
- Paget's disease, chemotherapy treatment, and history of radiation are risk factors.
- Typically seen in younger adults but may be seen in patients over 40 years of age.
- Occurs at metaphyseal regions of long bones.
- May have lung metastasis at time of diagnosis. Presents as bone pain with, at times, associated palpable mass.
- Plain films may demonstrate sunburst sign (cortical destruction) and Codman's triangle.
- Treatment includes
    - Neoadjuvant chemotherapy
    - excision with 4 cm margins
    - high-grade lesions may require limb reconstruction or amputation.

Ewing's Sarcoma

- From neuroectoderm
- Typically seen in children aged 5–15 years
- Symptoms include fever, malaise, edema, and pain
- Chromosome 11-22 translocation
- May be seen in pelvis, femur, diaphysis of humerus
- radiographs demonstrate onion skinning.
- Treatments include chemotherapy, radiation therapy, and resection.

Rhabdomyosarcoma

- Typically seen in children between 2 to 5 YOA or 15-19 YOA
- Most common pediatric sarcoma
- Starts as mesenchyme but differentiates into skeletal muscle
- Presents as a palpable mass
- May be a history of trauma in area but this is red herring
- Perform incisional biopsy; image with MRI and CT
- Treatment includes chemotherapy and wide local excision

Pediatric Surgery

Medial umbilical ligament is the obliterated (remnant) umbilical artery

Median umbilical ligament is the obliterated urachus

Shunts and fetal circulation

- Blood enters fetal circulation via the one umbilical vein (eventually becomes the ligamentum teres hepatis contained in falciform in adult)
- Umbilical vessels are 2 arteries and one vein only
- Then blood bypasses liver via ductus venosus (in adult becomes ligamentum venosum) and enters IVC
- Goes to right atrium and, because right sided pressures are greater than left, enters left atrium via foramen ovale. Most flow goes this way.
- Any blood that enters pulmonary circulation instead of going through foramen ovale eventually enters the left pulmonary artery and leaves via the ductus arteriosus (becomes ligamentum arteriosum in the adult) and then enters descending aorta
- Most flow / cardiac output leaves fetus via the umbilical arteries to undergo oxygenation at placenta before returning via that umbilical vein (again becomes ligamentum teres hepatis in adult)

Gut development

- Foregut
  Structures that derive from foregut include lungs, esophagus, stomach, pancreas, and portion of duodenum proximal to ampulla.

- Midgut
  Gives rise to structures including duodenum distal to ampulla, small bowel, and large bowel to distal 1/3 of transverse colon

- Hindgut
  Distal 1/3 of transverse colon to anal canal derives from hindgut.

Peds vital signs

- 8 years to adult
  RR 12-20, HR 60-100, SBP 90-140

- 1 to 8 years
  RR 15-30, HR 80-100, SBP 80-110

- 1 month to 1 year old
  RR 25-50, HR 100-140, SBP 70-95

- newborn to one month
  RR 40-60, HR 120-160, SBP > 60

Prematurity is birth at < 37 weeks

Low birthweight definition is less that 2.5 kg at birth

Higher alkaline phosphatase in children compared to adults because children have growing bones. To tell whether alkaline phosphatase is from liver or bone on lab tests remember that "bone burns and liver lasts" meaning alkaline phosphatase from bone source is not stable at increased temperatures.

Pulmonary system

- Alveoli arise at approximately gestation week 24
- From 6 months to 6 years, infants breath mostly through their noses
- This system is not completely developed until around 8 years of age.

Renal System

- Remember that very little cardiac output goes to the kidneys in neonates. Only about 2-4%, where in adults approximately 25% of cardiac output goes to the kidneys.
- As a result of this and other factors, newborn kidneys are not as able to concentrate urine.
- Max concentration is approximately 500 milli-osmoles.
- Glomerular filtration rate (GFR) of full term baby is is approximately 2-4 mL per minute, and this increases by a factor of 5 to 10 in the first week of life.
- Adequate urine output for an infant is approximately 2-3mL per kilogram per hour.

Immune system

- Breast fed infant acquires IgA from breast milk
- IgG crosses placenta to provide maternally acquired immunity to fetus
- Infant immune system produces IgG eventually, but is slow to do so.
- Newborn immune system is also characterized by decreased complement fixation and polymorphonuclear neutrophil (PMN) function.

Fluid requirements

- Remember newborns have increased insensible volume loses compared to adults
- Also, newborns demonstrate physiologic diuresis during first week of life
- Holliday and Segar formula gives maintenance fluid rate for children
  - For first 10kg, 4mL per kg per hour
  - For second 10kg, 2 mL per kg per hour
  - For each kg after first 20kg, 1 mL per kg per hour
  - Example: maintenance rate requirement for 50 pound child:
    - 50 pounds (1 kg / 2.2 pounds) = 22.7 kg
    - 40 for first 10kg + 20 for second 10 kg + 1 times 2.7 for additional 2.7 kg = 62.7mL / hr maintenance fluid
- typically use D51/4NS for children for maintenance but there are options
- initial bolus for shock in pediatric trauma is 20mL/kg. May repeat. If patient remains / is unstable, give 10mL/kg PRBCs next.
  Best indicator of shock is tachycardia (see age appropriate vital signs listed above)

Nutritional requirements

- 18 years old to 10 years old
  50-60 kcal/kg/day (1.0 g protein/kg/day)

- 10 years old to 7 years old
  70 kcal/kg/day (1.0-1.5 g protein/kg/day)

- 3 years old to 6 months old
  100 kcal/kg/day (1.2-1.6 g protein/kg/day)

- Full term baby
  110-120 kcal/kg/day (2-2.5 g protein/kg/day)

- Preterm baby
  120-130 kcal/kg/day (3-4 g protein/kg/day)

Choanal atresia

- Posterior nares occlusion
- More common in twins
- Retractions related to respiratory distress (intermittent) seen
- Diagnosis made when unable to pass nasogastric tube beyond anterior nares
- Treatment is resection and postop stent to preserve patency

Thyroglossal duct cyst

- From ectodermal rests the persist after thyroid descends through area
- This is the most frequent congenital anomaly of the neck
- Over 50% may not be diagnosed until adulthood...but remember, a biopsy of a node in lateral neck that returns as "normal thyroid tissue" or "ectopic thyroid tissue" is PAPILLARY THRYOID CANCER, NOT thyroglossal duct cyst
- Thyroglossal duct cyst is midline neck mass below the level of hyoid bone that does move with swallowing. It is NOT lateral. (Unlike the biopsy situation above.)
- Mass moves up toward head when tongue is protruded
- See a midline neck mass in pediatric patient? Think thyroglossal duct cyst and evaluate for that. See a lateral neck mass in pediatric population? Think brachial cleft cyst. (Next section.)
- Treatment is Sistrunk procedure which involves removing the cyst AND the associated tract up to the base of the tongue AND the central portion of the hyoid bone. Otherwise there is a papillary thyroid cancer risk if entire tract not excised.

Anomalies of Branchial Cleft

- Sinuses, cysts, or fistulas seen in lateral neck
- Most arise from second brachial cleft (90% arise from there)
- Typically see drainage from a small pit in the skin associated with lower one-third of sternocleidomastoid
- Clear fluid from anterior neck pit is seen
- MRI or CT imaging demonstrates cystic mass in anterior neck
- Resection cyst and tract, note that tract may run between branches of carotid and extend to pharynx

Cystic hygroma

- Seen in posterior neck, axillae, and supraclavicular region
- Lymphatic lesion. Benign.
- Painless mass that transilluminates and is compressible
- prenatal ultrasound may make diagnosis
- CT and MRI demonstrate lesion and possibly deep extent into the chest / mediastinum
- Surgical excision or injection with sclerosing agent are treatment options
- If infected, treat infection and delay resection by approximately three weeks or until infection cleared

Torticollis

- 50-70% resolve by 8 months of age if untreated
- due to fetal position en utero or trauma to sternocleidomastoid (SCM) during birth
- during first several weeks of life, SCM contracture occurs
- clinical diagnosis, but imaging rules out other causes
- treatment is physical therapy

Tracheoesophageal fistula

- Seen in 0.2% of births
- 10% of cases are associated with VACTERL (Vertebral anomalies, Anorectal anomalies, Cardiac anomalies, Tracheo-Esophageal fistulas, Renal/radial anomalies, Limb anomalies) syndrome
- patients with associated esophageal atresia often present with drooling & inability to tolerate feeds
- patients with trachea-esophageal fistula, after eating, demonstrate respiratory distress and coughing after eating
- if maternal polyhydramnios seen then infant may have complete atresia
- failure to pass an NGT demonstrates all types except type E (aka H type) fistula
- bronchoscopy and esophagoscopy confirm diagnosis
- contrast imaging carries higher risk of pneumonitis and is rarely necessary
- Tracheoesophageal fistula is a risk factor for tracheomalacia
    - Tracheomalacia includes elliptical rings at trachea instead of c shaped ones
    - "dying spell" is most common sign. Also may see failure to ween from vent. Also see wheezing.
    - Most resolve at 1-2 years old.
    - If surgery is required, aortopexy is treatment. Suture aorta to posterior sternum to allow improved tracheal patency.

- Types
    - A type: esophageal atresia with no fistula. Looks like portion of esophagus is "missing".
    - B type: looks like A type EXCEPT proximal portion of esophagus has a fistula to trachea.
    - C type: looks like A type EXCEPT distal portion of esophagus has fistula to trachea.
    - D type: looks like A type EXCEPT proximal AND distal portion of esophagus each have fistula to trachea.
    - E type: unlike A type, esophagus is in continuity although it may be narrow. Fistula present to trachea. ALSO CALLED H type because it looks like a letter H.
- Surgical intervention includes extrapleural thoracotomy. Staying in extrapleural position avoids pleural contamination if post op leak occurs. Fistula is divided and primary reanastamosis of esophagus is performed. Long gap atresia and (may be seen in A type) and pure atresia may need staged repair over time. Type E (H type) may be repaired via neck incision.

Congenital lobar emphysema

- Air trapping gives lung hyperexpansion
- May develop hemodynamic instability for same reasons seen with tension pneumothorax
- Typically left upper lobe affected
- Bronchus is blocked owing to cartilaginous malformation
- Mediastinal shift seen with eventual respiratory failure
- Typically seen in left upper or right middle love
- Often no symptoms at birth
- Diagnose with CT or pCXR
- Perform lobectomy of affected area
- Beware: do NOT diagnose congenital lobar emphysema as a pneumothorax because placing a chest tube into the area of congenital lobar emphysema patients may lead to decompensation

Congenital cystic adenomatoid malformation

- Communicating cysts at terminal bronchioles level
- Cysts become infected and also trap air
- May be seen on prenatal ultrasound and may spontaneously regress
- Range of presentations from severe respiratory distress at birth to asymptomatic
- CXR or CT to diagnose
- Treatment is resection as there is thought that these may lead to malignant regeneration

Bronchogenic cyst

- These cysts are typically extra-pulmonary cysts that arise from bronchial tissue and cartilage wall.
- On occasion, may be intra-pulmonary in position.
- Mediastinal mass filled with milky appearing fluid
- Have malignant potential and cause compression of nearby structures. May also become infected.
- Treatment includes resection of cyst

Pulmonary sequestration

- Does NOT communicate with trachea or bronchi
- Most commonly presents with infection
- Arterial supply is from systemic circulation
  - Most commonly from thoracic aorta
  - May be abdominal aorta via inferior pulmonary ligament
- Venous drainage varies with type of pulmonary sequestration
  - Intralobar is most common type, drains through pulmonary veins
    Treatment is lobectomy
  - Extralobar drains via azygous veins (systemic circulation)
    - Seen more commonly in males
    - Diagnosed earlier owing to other anomalies seen in these patients
    - Treatment is excision of lesion
    - Exam may yield a bruit over affected site
    - Typically L lower lobe affected
- CTA or MRA imaging may demonstrate systemic systemic blood flow to tissue
- May require embolization if intra-lesion shunt is compromising hemodynamic status
- These arteries typically traverse inferior pulmonary ligament. Care is taken to identify and ligate these vessels in the chest order to avoid retraction of the vessels beneath the diaphragm which results in uncontrolled bleeding. Ligate arterial supply first, then lobectomy.

Childhood mediastinal masses by position

- Most common lesions are neurogenic tumors
  - Posterior mediastinum
    - Neurofibroma
    - Ganglioneuroma
    - Meningioma
    - Neuroblastoma
  - Middle mediastinum
    - Lymphoma
    - Teratoma
    - Bronchogenic cyst
    - Cardiogenic cyst
  - Anterior mediastinum
    - Lymphoma
    - Germ cell tumor, eg teratoma
    - Thymoma
    - Thyroid cancer

Congenital diaphragm hernia

- The big problem is pulmonary hypoplasia that results from the herniation of abdominal viscera into thoracic cavity
- Unfortunately, even though commonly one side is herniated, dysfunction is seen in BOTH lungs.
- 1/3000 live births, and may have autosomal dominant or recessive inheritance at times
- hernias on right may allow herniation of liver and small bowel
- hernias on left more typically involve colon and small bowel
- most common presentation involves respiratory distress in first few hours of life in association with enlarged "barrel" chest and scaphoid abdomen. In some causes bowel sounds may be heard over chest wall
- in utero may be diagnosed with ultrasound
- pCXR may show NGT in chest and bowel in chest
- 80% of patients have additional anomalies, so remember to evaluate other organs (often done during repair)
- delay procedure to repair until pulmonary hypertension resolves
- options for repair include approach via abdomen or chest and primary or mesh repair
- depending upon severity of pulmonary issues, patient may require extracorporeal membrane oxygenation (ECMO) temporarily
- Morgagni's hernia
  - Rarely seen
  - Anterior location
- Bochdalek's hernia
  - More common than Morgagni's
  - Posterior location
- survival is 50% and as high as 80% in centers that specialize more specifically in this condition

Pyloric stenosis

- Much greater incidence in males (4:1 vs females)
- Additional factors include family history of disease and being a firstborn
- Presents as nonbilious projectile vomitus and inability to tolerate feeds at approximately 3-6 weeks of age
- Classic physical exam sign is olive sign in upper abdomen
- Lab tests demonstrate hypochloremic, hypokalemic metabolic acidosis
- Findings on ultrasound of pylorus with of > 4mm muscle thickness, channel length > 17mm, diameter > 14mm all consistent with pyloric stenosis diagnosis
- First correct hypovolemia and electrolyte disturbances
    - Normal saline first
    - Then D5 NS with 10 mEq K for maintenance
    - Do NOT do initial resus with potassium containing fluids owing to risk of hyperkalemia developing quickly in these patients
    - Use D5 fluid when possible because young children do not perform gluconeogenesis as well as adults and so require that D5
- After those are corrected, perform pyloromyotomy
    - Proximal extent is circular muscle of stomach
    - If leak or concerned about violating mucosa, suture initial myotomy closed, rotate pylorus to posterior portion, and perform myotomy at that location

Choledochal cyst

- Dilation of biliary tree from birth with significant malignant potential
- While common in Asian populations, this is rare in the United States
- Seen more commonly in females. 4:1 female to male ratio.
- Classifications
    - Type 1
        - Most common type. Long segment of duct is dilated.
        - Treatment is total cyst excision.
    - Type 2
        - One diverticulum of ductal system. Extrahepatic duct only effected.
        - Treatment is total cyst excision.
    - Type 3
        - Confined to portion of bile duct that traverses the duodenal wall
        - Treatment is sphincterotomy and transduodenal excision
    - Type 4A
        - Multiple cysts. Both intra and extrahepatic ducts involved.
        - Partial hepatectomy if localized to one lobe of liver. If both lobes, transplant.
    - Type 4B
        - Multiple cysts. Involves extrahepatic ducts only.
        - Treatment is cyst excision
    - Type 5
        - Many cysts. Involves intrahepatic ducts only. Also known as Caroli's disease.
        - Partial hepatectomy if localized to one lobe of liver. If both lobes, transplant.
        - If cysts remain unresected, complications include pancreatitis, cholangitis, obstructive jaundice, and cholangiocarcinoma
        - Ultrasound may provide diagnosis prenatally
        - CT and MRI imaging provide additional information. MRCP is useful to demonstrate anatomy.

Biliary atresia

- Progresses to hepatic fibrosis
- Affects extrahepatic bile ducts
- Affects 0.005% of infants (1/20,000 incidence)
- Possibly a result of immune response to viral infection
- 60% of cases are NOT associated with other conditions
- of 40% that ARE associated with other conditions, there are many different associations including polysplenia, preduodenal portal vein, ventricular septal defects, and situs inversus.
- Presentation includes clay color stools and jaundice that does not resolve by two weeks. Also failure to thrive owing in part to malabsorption.
- Conjugated hyperbilirubinemia is seen
- HIDA (hepatobiliary iminodiacetic acid) scan demonstrates tracer uptake but no excretion into duodenum. (Test is sensitive but not specific for biliary atresia.)
- ERCP and ultrasound assist with evaluating and ruling out other potential causes of biliary obstruction
- Liver biopsy indicates obstructive (not hepatocellular) cause of stasis
- Kasai procedure (hepatoportoenterostomy) is treatment. Gallbladder and all ductal tissue up to level of liver capsule is resected. Roux limb of bowel anastamosed to ducts at level of liver capsule.
- Approximately 1/3 of Kasai patients die before transplant, 1/3 eventually receive a transplant, and for 1/3 Kasai is curative. (Obviously approximately 2/3 of Kasai patients will eventually need transplant whether they actually receive one or not.)

Congenital pancreatic variants

- Annular pancreas
  - Results from incomplete or absent rotation of the ventral pancreatic bud
  - Causes duodenal obstruction
  - Do NOT resect any portion of the pancreas
  - Bypass the area with gastrojejunostomy or roux limb or some other option
- Pancreatic divisum
  - Failure of fusion of dorsal duct (Santorini duct) with ventral duct (Wirsung duct)
  - Surprisingly common. Affects 10% of the population.
  - Remember that Santorini is the small duct ("Santorini is Small.")
  - Pancreas may appear grossly to be one whole organ, but ERCP / MRCP demonstrates non-fusion of ducts. That is still considered divisum because whether or not the ducts are fused is the criteria for divisum...NOT the appearance of the gland.
  - Responsible for <1% of cases of pancreatitis. But when other options are ruled out, need to look to congenital causes.
  - Causes recurrent pancreatitis because small duct inadequately drains pancreas.
  - Treated via sphincteroplasty of the MINOR duodenal papilla where the small duct enters duodenum. Another less common option is Puestow procedure.

Malrotation

- Some surgeons call this condition "non-rotation" because it's failure of 270 counterclockwise rotation of midgut. (It's incomplete rotation.)
- May result in volvulus.
- Rotation normally occurs during 6th week of embryonic development.
- 90% are symptomatic at 1 year of age
  However, some do make it to adulthood without symptoms and it's estimated that approximately 1% of adults demonstrate non-rotation to some degree. It is often not appreciated on CT scans in adults and goes unnoticed when adults with non-rotation undergo CT for other reasons.
- Presents with bilious vomiting and failure to thrive. However, again, older children may have generalized abdominal pain.
- Children with bilious vomiting need emergent UGI to rule out malrotation
- Test to diagnose is UGI with SBFT demonstrates duodenum that does not cross midline (duodenal sweep does not cross midline).
- If any question of volvulus, requires immediate operation with detorsion of volvulus (counter clockwise rotation of bowel), placement of small bowel on patient's right and colon on patient's left, division of Ladd's bands, and appendectomy. (Entire procedure is Ladd's procedure.) Remember "Ladd's bands" may cause duodenal obstruction. They originate from R retroperitoneum. These are relieved as part of Ladd's procedure.

Intestinal Atresia

- Atresia is due to mesenteric infarcts
- Inability to tolerate feeds, bilious emesis
- Usually does not have distension
- Jejunum is common location but patient may have multiple sites
- Often perform rectal biopsy too to rule out Hirschprung's pre-op
- Double bubble sign on xray (dilated stomach and duodenum)
- Treated with bypass, eg duodenoduodenostomy or duodenojejunostomy

Intestinal Stenosis

- Due to failure of duodenum to recanalize
- 20% of patients with duodenal stenosis also have Down's syndrome
- similar to intestinal atresia in these respects:
  - Inability to tolerate feeds, bilious emesis
  - Usually does not have distension
  - Double bubble sign on xray (dilated stomach and duodenum)
  - Treated with bypass, eg duodenoduodenostomy or duodenojejunostomy

Omphalocele

- Occurs because umbilical sac does not close. Umbilical sac is normally involved in routine developmental intestinal herniation.
- Hernia contents include large or small bowel (or both), stomach, and even solid viscera (eg liver)
- Has peritoneal sac with cord attached
- High incidence (85%) of cases involve associated abnormalities. Most common abnormality is cardiovascular.
- Associated with Beckwith-Wiedemann Syndrome (macroglossia, macrosomia, and omphalocele)
- May have cloacal exstrophy
- Diagnosed typically with prenatal ultrasound
- First, check for associated anomalies. Then, treatment is abdominal closure (staged with silo or primary).
- GI abnormality most commonly associated: malrotation
- Prognosis is worse than gastroschisis because of associated abnormalities.
- Pentalogy of Cantrell
    - cardiac defects
    - Pericardium defects at diaphragmatic pericardium
    - Sternal cleft / portion of sternum absent
    - Septum transversum defectus (portion of diaphragm absence)
    - omphalocele

Gastroschisis

- Umbilical sac DOES close but para-umbilical hernia (right side) occurs
- Due to rupture of umbilical vein in utero
- There is NO sac over defect / organs in area. So organs are exposed to amnion etc. Bowel and other contents are stiffened.
- Contents of hernia is typically small bowel unlike omphalocele where many other organs may be involved.
- Associated anomalies are much less common than omphalocele. Only seen in 10% of gastroschisis cases. May be associated with intestinal atresia and Hirschprung's disease. Yes, malrotation may still be present as in omphalocele but much less commonly seen.
- Typically diagnosed with prenatal ultrasound.
- Treatment is abdominal closure (either primary or staged with silo). Cover bowel with moist towel and prevent venous obstruction from mesenteric kinking.

Umbilical hernia

- Linea alba doesn't close resulting in defect
- many close by approx. age 3
- seen in premature infants more commonly
- seen in African American children more commonly
- If not closed by age five should repair. Also repair if incarcerations. Another indication is VP shunt presence because if an issue occurs with hernia will be a problem with shunt contamination. Also effluent from shunt may worsen hernia over time without repair.

Meconium Ileus

- Seen in > 10% of cystic fibrosis patients
- Is due to thickened mucus secreted by small intestine which leads to small bowel obstruction.
- Bilious emesis, failure to pass meconium postnatally, and abdominal distension are seen.
- Ground glass or soap bubble seen on xray owing to meconium mixed with air (Neuhauser's sign)
- Clinical diagnosis
- Initial treatment is NG decompression and hydration. Then gastroview enema. This resolves 80% of cases.
- If this fails, ex lap with enterotomy and evacuation performed.
- Irrigation of mucosa with gastroview, saline, or acetylcysteine may be required. Appendectomy may also be performed owing to high risk of appendicitis in patients with cystic fibrosis.

Hirschprung's Disease

- Failure of neural crest cell migration resulting in absence of ganglion cells in Auerbach's plexus. This results in absence of peristalsis and distal bowel obstruction.
- RET proto-oncogene association
- 1 in 5000 births
- billions emesis, abdominal distension, and failure to pass meconium are typically seen
- rectal suction biopsy demonstrates absence of ganglion cells and makes diagnosis
- one or two-staged colectomy with resection of involved tissue and a pull-through procedure is treatment
- may see Hirschprung's colitis. Sometimes requires emergent colectomy. Is due to backup owing to issue with lacking plexus. Sepsis may be present. Rectal irrigation may be attempted to attempt to empty colon.

Imperforate Anus

- Defect in cloaca partitioning into rectum and urogenital sinus
- More commonly seen in males
- Association with VACTERL syndrome.
- Abnormalities seen ABOVE levator ani muscles (high anomalies) often to NOT exhibit ectopic opening on exam but may include fistula with urinary system
- Anomalies BENEATH level of levator muscles (low anomalies) typically show perineal opening in males and fistula to vagina in females. Sphincter anatomy is preserved in low lesions.
- Ultrasound may be useful to make diagnosis
- Fistula above levators are treated with colostomy and anal reconstruction with posterior sagittal anoplasty
- Beneath levators treated with posterior sagittal anoplasty and anal dilation

Necrotizing enterocolitis (NEC)

- Most common gastrointestinal emergency among neonates in the ICU
- Overally mortality approximately 10%
- Infections, hypoxia, prematurity, enteral feeding, and use of umbilical catheter each associated with NEC
- Bloody stools, ileus, feed intolerance, abdominal distension, ileus, abdominal wall erythema, and hemodynamic instability are all associated with NEC.
- Classic history is bloody stools after first feed
- Clinical diagnosis that abdominal xray confirms. May see free air, pneumatosis intestinalis, and / or portal venous air.
- Only ABSOLUTE indication for operation is free air
- Other indications to operate (in general) are relative indications and include: persistent acidosis, abdominal wall erythema, and persistent fixed loop of bowel on xray
- Uncomplicated NEC is managed medically with decompression, bowel rest, fluid resuscitation and antibiotics.
- Operative treatment includes laparotomy and resection of gangrenous and any perforated bowel. May use second look to re-eval any questionable areas. Bring up ostomies
- Post op complications include sepsis, DIC, recurrence, and stricture.
- Mortality in those requiring surgery is approximately 60%
- Check barium enema to rule out stricture prior to ostomy reversal

Intussusception

- One portion of bowel telescopes into another
- Again…
    - The intussusCIPIENS is the part of the bowel that is the reCIPIENT of another piece.
    - The other part of the bowel involved is the intussusceptum
- Most cases in children are idiopathic (UNLIKE adult intussusception)
- highest incidence 3 months to 2 years
- most common cause is idiopathic. Other lead points include enlarged Peyer's patches, polyps, Meckel's, tumors, or duplication cysts.
- Currant jelly stools is classic description of associated stool. These are owing to vascular congestion but presence is NOT an indication for resection.
- Ileocecal junction is most common location
- Abdominal pain, currant jelly stools, and palpable abdominal mass triad (Classic triad) is present in less than 50%
- Air contrast enema is diagnostic and successful in treating 80% of cases
    - High perforation risk if you exceed these values with reduction attempt
        - Max column height (if barium enema used instead of air contrast) = 1 meter
        - Max pressure (air contrast enema) = 120 mm Hg
        - Go to OR if these values are reached after about an hour of attempts
- Recurrence rate is 15% are reduction with air contrast enema
- If contrast enema fails, patient requires open or laparoscopic reduction.
- Intussusceptum is milked from intussuscipiens, ischemic bowel is resected if present, and evaluation for pathologic lead point is performed.
- May require appendectomy if there is vascular compromise noted owing to occurrence at ileocecal junction with vascular compromise.
- Remember, in children lead points = inflamed Peyer's patch, lymphoma, Meckel's (most to least common) so benign lead point is most common. However, in adults, malignant lead point more common. So adult cases need to be treated with that in mind.

Meckel's Diverticulum

- Seen in 2% of the population, making it the most common congenital anomaly of the small intestine
- Due to persistent omphalomesenteric duct (vitelline duct)
- Classic "Rule of 2s": seen 2% of population, found 2 feet from ileocecal valve, 2% have symptoms, presentation typically by age 2, 2 types of mucosa (gastric and pancreatic)
- May present as drainage from umbilicus in children
- Three fourths are diagnosed before patient reaches ten years of age
- May present with bleeding, intussusception, volvulus, perforation, or obstruction
- Meckel's scan (technicium 99 pertechnetate scan) demonstrates gastric mucosa
- In the presence of symptoms, requires resection with small bowel anastomosis. Remember, ulceration of bowel occurs on the side opposite the Meckel's as secretions injury the bowel mucosa opposite the diverticulum. (Note that some advocate wedge resection of diverticulum with transverse closure of ileum.)
- Watch out. What you think may be appendicitis is sometimes in fact a Meckel's.

Pectus Excavatum

- Sternal & anterior chest wall deformity
- Decreased lung volumes and exercise tolerance noted
- Physical exam makes the diagnosis
- Nuss procedure is insertion of bar behind sternum and anterior to pericardium. Ectopy often seen on passing bar from one side of patient to the other anterior to heart and in retrosternal position.
- Ravitch procedure includes osteotomy of sternum with cartilage resection

Hydrocele

- Seen most commonly in preterm infants
- Nontender fluid collection in processus vaginalis
- A newborn's bowel will transilluminate as will fluid in the area, so transillumination is not useful to determine whether this represents an isolated hydrocele or hernia in the area
- Some hydroceles communicate with the peritoneal cavity, and those may change in size with position as fluid moves between scrotum and peritoneum.
- Non-communicating hydrocele's do not change in size with position. The differentiation between communicating and non-communicating is useful because non-communicating hydroceles will usually resolve on their own.
- Treatment for communicating hydrocele is to resect and ligate processes vaginalis.

Testicular Torsion

- Bell-clapper deformity occurs when gubernaculum testis does not tether the testis properly so it is only tethered on one side and may torse within the tunica vaginalis. It looks like a bell clapper because it "hangs" only on one side.
- This torsion results in impaired blood flow.
- Loss of ipsilateral cremasteric reflex is seen because the cremasteric muscle is shortened and swollen owing to the torsion.
- This is diagnosed clinically; however, an ultrasound may evaluate blood flow to the testis.
- Treatment is operative detorsion with orchiopexy BILATERALLY because the bell clapper deformity may be present bilaterally.

Cryptorchidism

- Diagnosed by exam when testis not present in scrotum
- May confirm diagnosis with MRI if unsure
- Usually examine patient again at 6 months because many testes will descend by then.
- Treatment includes placing testes in scrotum and fixation in scrotal pouch
- One third of patients acquire testicular involution by 2 years of age if untreated
- Also a risk factor for germ cell cancer and infertility

Neuroblastoma

- Typically arises from adrenal gland
- From neural crest cells
- So elevated VMA, metanephrines, catecholamines and HVA are seen. May cause hypertension in peds patients.
- Doesn't invade vascular structures. Surrounds and encases them.
- Most common extracranial solid tumor in children less than 2 years old
- Wilm's tumor is most common solid tumor in children older than two years old.
- Multiple non-specific abdominal complaints may be associated with lesion, but often asymptomatic
- Peri-orbital ecchymosis, palpable mass, and opsoclonus myoclonus may be seen on exam.
- Age at diagnosis is VERY important: in children less than one year old, tumors are often lower stage AND spontaneously regress. In children greater than one year old, tumors typically are more advanced in stage and prognosis is much worse.
- If patient has mets, neuron specific enolase (NSE) will be elevated.
- In some children less than 6 months old with a small lesion, even with mets to liver, skin, and bone, there is a very favorable prognosis.
- neuron specific enolase, LDH, > 3 copies N-myc gene, aneuploidy in tumors...all give worse prognosis

- Staging
  - Stage 1
    Localized tumor with complete excision

  - Stage 2A
    Localized tumor with incomplete excision

  - Stage 2B
    Localized tumor with incomplete excision and positive ipsilateral nodes

  - Stage 3
    Unresectable tumor that crosses midline and involves contralateral nodes

  - Stage 4
    Distant lymph node involvement and primary tumor

  - Stage 4S
    Skin, bone marrow, and liver involvement as well as localized tumor (seen in children less than 1 year of age only)

Wilms' Tumor

- Due to a deletion on chromosome 11
- Syndromes associated with Wilm's tumor
  - Denys-Drash syndrome
    Wilm's, nephropathy, intersex disorders
  - Hemihypertrophy
  - Beckwith Wiedemann syndrome
    gigantism, visceromegaly, macroglossia, omphalocele
  - WAGR
    Wilm's, mental retardation, aniridia, GU malformations
- This is the most common malignant renal lesion of childhood.
- Approximately 10% are bilateral
- Typically diagnosed at 2-3 years of age
- Classic history is mass noticed by parents during bathing
- May present with L sided varicocele, abdominal / flank pain, hematuria or hypertension
- US may be used to determined whether IVC invasion or renal vein invasion is present. CT chest and abdomen are performed to rule out bilateral lesion, metastasis, and confirm diagnosis.

- Wilm's tumor staging
  - Stage 1
    Limited to kidney and completely excised
  - Stage 2
    Tumor NOT limited to kidney, but completely excised
  - Stage 3
    Residual lesion with metastases but non-hematogenous metastases
  - Stage 4
    Hematogenous metastases
  - Stage 5
    Tumor is bilateral
- Prognosis is typically based on GRADE
- Worse prognosis with sarcomatous or anaplastic types
- Treatments is excision including nephrectomy with examination of contralateral kidney and neoadjuvant chemo Vincristine, doxyrubicin, actinomycin are used
- Nephrectomy generally cures 90%
- Radiation may be added for stage 3 disease
- If disease is bilateral, often conserve as much kidney function as possible with partial nephrectomy.

Hepatoblastoma

- Typically affects males
- Seen in children less than three years old
- Associated with familial adenomatous polyposis and Beckwith-Wiedemann syndrome
- Often no symptoms other than slowly increasing abdominal girth
- Owing to HCG production, precocious puberty may be present
- Make diagnosis with biopsy and MRI
- Alpha fetoprotein elevation is seen in 90%
- Cisplatin and doxyrubicin are used as adjuvant of neoadjuvant therapy along with resection
- Approximately 75% of cases are curable

Hemangioma

- Grow quickly during first 6-12 months of life, then dissipate
- Observe initially because most resolve by 8 years of age
- If lesion is in a spot that inhibits function (eyelid for example), grows uncontrollably, or persists after age 8 treat with oral steroids
- May use laser or resect if other treatments not effective

Abdominal Wall, Hernias, & Mesh

From deep to superficial, the muscular layers of the abdominal wall spell TIE. TIE = Tranverse abdominus, Internal oblique, and External oblique.

Camper's and Scarpa's "fascia" are superficial to the external oblique, and the peritoneum is deep to the tranverse abdominus. Camper's is fatty tissue and is superficial to Scarpa's. Scarpa's fascia is a deeper and more fibrous layer.

The Arcuate Line of Douglas is a line created by how the muscles of the abdomen are situated. Inferiorly, the Internal oblique fascia layers are completely anterior to the rectus abdominal muscle. So 2 layers (internal oblique and external oblique) fascia are anterior the rectus. Superiorly in the abdomen, the internal oblique fascia splits and encompasses the rectus abdominus. So only one and one half layers of fascia are anterior to the rectus (one half the internal oblique fascia and the external oblique fascia). The fact that the abdominal wall abruptly transitions from 2 layers anterior to rectus inferiorly to 1.5 layers (more superiorly) gives the appearance of a line on the abdomen. That line is the Arcuate Line of Douglas.

MANY named abdominal hernias exist. Here are some of the classic ones

- Lumbar hernias
  - Grynfeltt's hernia passes through the superior lumbar triangle
  - Petit's hernia occurs through the inferior lumbar triangle (bounded by the iliac crest, external oblique, and the latissimus dorsi)
- Spigelian hernia
  - High risk of incarceration (20%)
  - Requires repair
  - Hernia occurs in the space lateral to the posterior rectus sheath to the medial portion of the tranverse abdominus
  - This is through the linea semilunaris
- Epigastric hernia occurs through the linea alba
- Littre's hernia is a hernia that contains a Meckel's diverticulum.
- Pantaloon hernia (so named because it looks like pantaloons) occurs when an inguinal hernia has both a direct and indirect component that is restricted by the epigastric vessels so that it is similar in appearance to a pair of pantaloons.
- Obturator hernia seen in elderly women and is associated with Howship-Romberg sign (pain at inner thigh with medial rotation). Bowel obstruction and medial, palpable thigh mass may be seen. Occurs through obturator foramen and so is medial and anterior to obturator nerve and vessels.
- Richter's hernia may yield bowel perforation WITHOUT obstruction. This occurs when only one portion of wall of bowel is within hernia and becomes ischemic / necrotic.

Umbilical hernias

- Childhood umbilical hernias are usually not repaired until approximately four years of age owing to high rate of spontaneous closure.
- Risk factors for congenital umbilical hernias include
  - African American race
  - Prematurity
- Risk factors for developing an umbilical hernia include
  - Female gender
  - Any condition that increases intra-abdominal pressure
    Eg pregnancy, obesity, cirrhosis / ascites, intra-abdominal mass
- Umbilical hernias in adults rarely close spontaneously
- Are due to a defect in the linea alba at the level of the umbilicus
- Do not repair umbilical hernias in patients with cirrhosis and ascites unless there is already an ascites leak / skin necrosis over the hernia or obvious incarcerated bowel with a concern for strangulation. This is because post-operative ascites leak from an elective umbilical hernia repair may lead to worsening liver failure and decompensation.

Incisional hernia

- Risk factors include increasing age, wound infection post op, poor nutrition, tobacco use, corticosteroid usage, emergent repair, poor closure technique, immunosuppression.
- Usually seen in first post op year
- 10-20% of patients who have an abdominal procedure
- Bulge noted on exam. Maybe painful or painless. May have incarcerated structure or none.
- Primary repair is associated with a greater recurrence rate than mesh repair, however some patients are not candidates for mesh repair.
- Multiple approaches for repair are possible.

Femoral hernias

- 15% are bilateral
- Although these are more commonly seen in women than men, inguinal hernia is still the most common hernia in women.
- Higher risk of incarceration (and strangulation) than inguinal hernia because hernia orifice (neck) is more narrow.
- Exam demonstrates a bulge at the upper medial thigh and inferior to inguinal ligament.
- Operative repair is indicated owing to incarceration risk. McVay repair is typically performed. If strangulation present, requires emergent repair.
- Requires Cooper's ligament repair (McVay does this)
- Lateral boundary is femoral vein, medial is lacunar ligament, anterior is inguinal ligament, posterior is Cooper's ligament
- May need to divide inguinal ligament to reduce bowel

Inguinal hernia

- Most common type of hernia (75%)
- 50% are indirect, 25% are direct, approximately 25% are both.
- Much more common in men
- Right side more common than left
- Heavy exercise, ascites, and any condition that increases intra-abdominal pressure is risk factor
- Indirect hernia
  - Indirect hernias result from a patent processus vaginalis and arise lateral to Hesselbach's triangle
  - Protusion of abdominal contents through the internal ring
  - Hernia sac is anteromedial to the cord
- Direct hernia
  - Passes through weakness in transversalis fascia
  - Protrude directly through Hesselbach's triangle
- "Sliding hernia" is the term given to inguinal hernias in which abdominal contents slide into hernia sac…eg cecum, ovary, appendix, etc.
- incarceration and strangulation of contents requires emergent repair
- nerves in inguinal region and associated lumbar levels
  - genitofemoral nerve from L1 and L2
  - iliohypogastric from T12 and L1
  - ilioinguinal nerve from L1
- late hernia recurrences are felt to be caused by loss of fascial strength and early recurrences are felt to be due to inadequate repairs

- Repair techniques include
  - Laparoscopic repairs
    - TAP (TransAbdominal Preperitoneal)
    - TEP (Totally ExtraPeritoneal) approach
    - laparoscopic inguinal hernia repair should be considered for inguinal hernia repair when bilateral of recurrent hernias are encountered. Also for femoral repair.
  - Open repair (primary)
    - Care is taken to avoid sutures in pubic tubercle which may cause osteitis and pain.
    - Bassini repair includes inguinal floor reconstruction with approximation of the transversalis fascia, shelving edge of inguinal ligament, and conjoint tendon. High ligation of sac is performed. Primary repair.
    - Shouldice repair is primary repair using running suture to re-construct floor. Includes high ligation of the sac. Primary repair.
    - McVay repair is a primary repair where closure involves Cooper's ligament.
  - Open repair with mesh
    - Avoid prosthetic mesh if infection present
    - Lichtenstein repair involves mesh reconstruction of the inguinal floor with mesh.
    - Stoppa repair "plug and patch"
- Complications
  - Recurrence
  - Wound infection
  - Ischemic orchitis & testicular atrophy
    Caused by thrombosis of spermatic vessels during dissection or vessel disruption
  - Urinary retention is the most common complication
  - Nerve injury
    - Signs include loss of cremasteric reflex and sensation to penis, scrotum, and medial thigh (ilioinguinal nerve) and sometimes PAIN
      - Pain usually due to compression of ilioinguinal nerve
      - Local infiltration (lidocaine) at ASIS with lidocaine can be diagnostic and therapeutic
    - Loss of sensation to lower abdomen and inguinal area (iliohypogastric nerve)
    - Insensate upper lateral thigh (femoral branch) or loss of sensation and cremasteric motor function (genital branch)
    - Placement of staples or tacking mesh lateral to femoral vessels and below iliopubic tract may injure lateral cutaneous, femoral branch of genitofemoral, or femoral nerves.
- When repairing an inguinal hernia in children, for patients in whom bilateral inguinal hernias are suspected, contralateral exploration is performed.
- In children, high ligation of the hernia sac is sufficient repair for indirect inguinal hernia.

Inguinal hernia anatomy

- Superficial (external) ring: from external oblique. This is the "exit" of the inguinal canal
- Deep (internal) ring: from transveralis (transverse abdominus) fascia. This is the "entrance" of internal ring.
- Gimbernat's (aka lacunar) ligament: portion of inguinal ligament that joins inguinal ligament at pubic tubercle to the pectineal line at pubis
- Poupart's (aka inguinal) ligament: from external oblique and connects anterior superior iliac spine (ASIS) to the pubic tubercle
- Iliopubic tract arises from pectineal line and deep to the inguinal ligament
- Cooper's (pectineal) ligament: from thickening of pectineal line and extends from the lacunar ligament
- Conjoint tendon: arises from the internal oblique and transverse abdominus
- Retzius' space is the preperitoneal space behind pubic symphysis. Laparoscopic hernia repairs are performed here.
- Hesselbach's triangle is created by the inguinal ligament inferiorly, epigastric vessels laterally, and rectus sheath medially.
- Contents of inguinal canal include round ligament or spermatocord with genital branch of genitofemoral nerve, cremaster muscle, vas deferens, testicular artery, pampiniform plexus and ilioinguinal nerve (superior to cord).

Vascular

Poiseuille's (pronounced "paw-zoy") law

- This is why short, wide IVs give better flow than central lines. Central lines have longer length and higher resistance.
- Flow is related to the radius of the tube TO THE FOURTH POWER (!)
- Flow is inversely related to length

Bernoulli principle

Indicates that, as the diameter of a blood vessel decreases (stenosis) blood flow increases and blood pressure DECREASES.

Laplace's law

- Tension in wall of vessel increases as intravascular pressure increases and vessel diameter increases.
- Tension in wall is directly proportional to pressure times radius of vessel
- So when it comes to aneurysms
    - Timing of operation to repair should be based on diameter of aneurysm because diameter indicates rupture risk
    - Decreasing blood pressure (eg HTN control) decreases risk of rupture

Layers of arterial vessel (inner to outer) spell IMA: tunica Intima, tunica Media, tunica Adventitia (or externa)

- Tunica intima is formed by an elastic basement membrane and a single layer of endothelial cells
- Tunica media is smooth muscle and elastic tissue
- Tunica adventitia is collagen

The most common congenital hypercoagulable disorder is activated protein C resistance, while smoking is the most common acquired hypercoagulable disorder.

Arteries under systemic pressure are more muscular than pulmonary vessels or systemic veins.

Veins function as "capacitance vessels"; they have the capacity to distend much more than arteries when subjected to increased volume without large changes in pressure.

Atherosclerosis progression includes injury to endothelium, macrophage accumulation, macrophages accumulate lipid (and are called "foam cells"). These foam cells become fatty streaks and smooth muscle increases in the area. More endothelial disruption is seen, followed by atheroma formation. A fibrous plaque is formed. This becomes a complex plaque, and then the complex plaque ruptures.

Segmental pressure measurement is the term given for the measurement of systolic blood pressure at sites along the extremities. A decrease in systolic blood pressure by > 20mmHg helps identify site of stenosis / occlusion.

The Ankle-brachial Index (ABI) is the ratio of the systolic blood pressure at the ankle to the systolic blood pressure at the upper arm.

- ABI > 1 = normal
- ABI 0.5-1 = moderate disease
  ABI 0.5-0.7 = Claudication
- ABI < 0.5 = severe disease
  - ABI 0.3 – 0.5 = rest pain
  - ABI < 0.3 = gangrene

Pulse volume recording (plethysmography) is used to assess whether there is (or is not) pulsatile blood flow in an area. It's useful in patients with calcified vessels because it does not depend on vessel compressibility. So it may be used in patients with calcified vessels.

Internal Carotid artery disease

- Presenting signs and symptoms
  - Carotid bruit (most common)
  - TIA or ophthalmic deficit (lasting < 24 hours)
    Note that TIAs are more usually due to emboli instead of low flow
  - CVA (ischemic stroke)
- Velocity is increased with narrowing at lumen. Severity of narrowing is determined by velocity as measured on Doppler ultrasound. Other tests such as CTA and MRA are adjuncts.

- Carotidendarterectomy (CEA) removes atherosclerotic plaque at carotid bifurcation. (Actually intima and portion of media are removed.)
- Acute stroke symptoms post CEA. Typically means return to OR asap to check for intimal flap. Rare exceptions exist. Some surgeons perform routine intra-op ultrasound to demonstrate no flap is present before leaving OR. These surgeons may elect not to return to OR even if stroke signs present post op. However, generally speaking stroke symptoms post CEA mean emergent return to OR.
- Pseudoaneurysm post op: drape and prep before intubation. Then intubate and repair. Presents as pulsatile mass after CEA with bleeding
- New-onset / worsening HTN post op CEA: caused by injury to carotid body. 20% of patients have this post op. Treatment is nipride so that area does not bleed.
- Mandibular branch of facial nerve injury. Corner of mouth is affected when patient smiles.
- MI is the most common cause of non-stroke related complications post CEA.
- Restenosis rate after CEA is 15%
- Indications vary based on presence or absence of carotid ulcer on imaging, percent stenosis, and presence or absence of symptoms.
- Establishing good distal endpoint is most important technical concern in procedure.

- If back pressure < 50mmHg, use shunt.
- Some surgeons use shunt every procedure.
- Vagus nerve injury presents as hoarseness from recurrent laryngeal nerve issues because recurrent laryngeal nerve comes from vagus
- Hypoglossal nerve injury presents with tongue pointing toward side of problem. Gives speech and chewing difficulty
- Glossopharyngeal nerve injury Rare and only seen with VERY high carotid dissections. Difficulty swallowing is noted.
- Ansa cervicalis injury...no significant symptoms. Ansa innervates neck strap muscles.
- If a recent CVA has occurred, CEA is recommended for 4-6 weeks after recovery.
- NASCET (North American Symptomatic Carotid Endarterectomy Trial): in symptomatic patients with 70% stenosis or greater, CEA significantly reduces risk of ipsilateral stroke.
- ACAS (Asymptomatic Carotid Atherosclerosis Study): 5 year stroke risk significantly decreased in asymptomatic patients with > 60% stenosis who are treated with CEA.
- If symptomatic with > 50% stenosis, repair. If asymptomatic with > 70% stenosis, repair.
- If internal carotid is completely occluded, do NOT repair (no benefit) but be careful to confirm that what duplex may say is completely occluded is NOT a very high grade stenosis. Further imaging is typically used despite duplex read as completely occluded in order to be sure there is no "string sign" of a very tight stenosis which carries a high stroke risk.
- If bilateral stenosis present, repair more narrow side first, and if same narrowing bilaterally repair the dominant side first.

Aortic Dissection

- Medial layer separates because of tear in intimal layer which allows blood to escape from vessel lumen into the area to cause further dissection
- Connective tissue disorders (eg Ehlers-Danlos, Marfan's) are risk factors
- Aortitis, pregnancy, cocaine use, amphetamine use, and bicuspid aortic valve are all risk factors
- Stanford classification (and DeBakey classification) are used to classify aortic dissection types. (See Cardiothoracic section for Stanford and DeBakey classifications.)
- Chest or back pain may be seen
- Heart failure, MI, CVA, aortic insufficiency, or other end-organ issues (eg renal failure) may be seen
- pCXR shows wide mediastinum
- imaging with MRI, CT, or TEE may be used to make diagnosis
- treatment includes beta blockade and nitroprusside for tight blood pressure control.
- Emergent operative intervention for type A dissection is indicated
    - Post op complications may include paralysis, MI, and extremity ischemia.
    - Mortality with operative intervention is approximately 15%.
    - Post op followup with yearly imaging is important because distal dilation and aneurysmal change may occur.
- Type B is managed non-operatively unless complication ensues.

Thoracic aortic aneurysm

- Less common that abdominal aortic aneurysm
- With Atherosclerotic type, wall remodeling and dilation are seen.
- Degenerative type may be due to infection (mycotic aneurysm)
- Degenerative type may also be due to collagen vascular disease (Marfan's, cystic medial degeneration, or Ehlers-Danlos)
- Often found incidentally on imaging studies
- If symptoms are present, it may be due to compressive effects *eg* compression of esophagus that gives dysphagia, stridor from tracheal compression, or vocal cord compression from recurrent laryngeal nerve issues. Obviously, rupture and leak may also produce symptoms.
- If asymptomatic & < 5cm, aggressively control blood pressure. (No surgery)
- If asymptomatic & > 6cm, operative repair.
- If enlarging > 1cm per year, operative repair.
- If symptomatic, repair.
- If patient has a collagen vascular / connective tissue disease, use a lower threshold for intervention.
- Cardiac bypass and median sternotomy are required for arch and ascending aneurysms.
- Aneurysms distal to left subclavian (descending aneurysms) are accessible via L thoracotomy with single lung ventilation. Preservation of spinal cord circulation is key.
- Endovascular repair is an option.
- Complications
    - Renal failure (approximately 5%)
    - Spinal cord ischemia (approximately 5%)
    - Esophageal injury
    - Vocal chord paralysis
    - Pulmonary failure
    - Death (5% for ascending repairs, higher for descending repairs)

Abdominal aortic aneurysm

- Tobacco use, family history, and HTN are some important risk factors.
- Supra-renal (proximal to renal arteries) aneurysms are uncommon. Leaks are typically seen posteriorly and laterally (to the left of midline). Risk of rupture is low until > 6-7cm.
- Mycotic (infected) aneurysms: previously present aneurysm become contaminated with bacteria.
- Indications for repair
    - Greater than 5.5 cm in a male or...
    - Greater than 5.0 in a female or...
    - Patients with higher rupture risk (eg COPD) or...
    - Those with mycotic aneuyrsms or...
    - Aneurysms enlarging more than 0.5-1 cm in a year should receive surgical repair.
- patients who do not meet those criteria should receive ultrasound followup
- Repair techniques include open repair or endovascular repair depending on certain factors.
  Endovascular repair techniques require an available area to "land" an endovascular prosthetic. In order to receive endovascular repair, the aorta needs to have minimal tortuousity (if any) and have an appropriate "neck", meaning a long enough distance between the take off of the renal arteries and the beginning of the aneurysm.
- Open repair techniques include transperitoneal and retroperitoneal approaches.

- Special situations in abdominal aortic aneurysm repair
    - For mycotic aneurysms, excise the aneurysm and perform extra-anatomic bypass. Patients require long term antibiotics. Staph infection is most common. Second most common is salmonella.
    - For supra-renal abdominal aortic aneurysms, use a thoraco-abdominal approach and plan to re-implant celiac axis and SMA.
    - In ruptured abdominal aortic aneurysms, first establish proximal control.
    - Ligate bleeding lumbars
    - Inflammatory aneurysms
        - Seen in males. NOT due to infection.
        - Remember: do not dissect duodenum from the aneurysm in cases of inflammatory abdominal aortic aneurysms.
        - 25% of cases, ureter is entrapped.
- Patients who undergo endovascular repair require yearly screening for endoleaks
    - Type 1 endoleak: This requires revision immediately. This is due to inadequate sealing at proximal or distal graft.
    - Type 2 endoleak: Repair ONLY if aneurysm is enlarging. This is due to continued flow through aneurysm due to collaterals.
    - Type 3 endoleak: Occurs when there is a leak between portions of a graft with independent / modular sections. This requires repair.
    - Type 4: due to porous graft. Treatment is observation. If that fails, nonporous stent is placed.
    - Type 5: aneurysm expansion without sign of leak from previous repair. Repeat EVAR or perform surgical repair.

- Periop complications include MI, renal failure, infection, erectile dysfunction, ischemia of the lower extremities, and colonic ischemia.
    - Colon ischemia is often due to inferior mesenteric artery hypoperfusion. If IMA back bleeding during procedure, collaterals are likely adequate and do not need to re-implant. If NO back bleeding from IMA, more likely to need re-implantation to perfuse colon.
    Confirm colon ischemia with colonoscopy, and if patient is septic / critically ill may require colectomy.
    - Paraplegia may occur post op due to aberrant Artery of Adamkiewicz (these usually originate well superior to level of abdominal aortic aneurysm).
    - Risk of mortality with open repair is approximately 2-4%.
- Graft infection is a later complication
    - Remember that staph epidermidis graft infection MUST be treated with vancomycin or linezolid. Although usual staph epi is susceptible to many antibiotics, staph epi acquired in the hospital that is in grafts is usually susceptible to vancomycin only or a similarly advanced antibiotic. (This fact is NOT institution specific and is seen around the country.)
    - Staph is most common, E.Coli is second most common.
    - However, graft infection may require extra-anatomic bypass and other adjuncts.
- Other complications present in a delayed fashion, including aorto-enteric fistula. (Rare complication—less that 1% of cases.)
  Graft erodes into duodenum. Graft is visible on EGD and that is used to confirm diagnosis in stable patient. May present with herald bleed. (Patient presents with brief episode of GI bleeding that stops.) Treatment includes excision of graft, repair of duodenum, antibiotics, and extra-anatomic bypass.

Mesenteric ischemia

- Typically seen in geriatric patients who have an underlying condition that predisposes them. (Typically afib.)
- Decreased flow and reperfusion injury are seen.
- Chronic mesenteric ischemia is typically caused by atherosclerosis of 2 or more visceral vessels and is most commonly seen in middle aged women with a decrease in flow over time. Presents as fear of eating ("food fear") that leads to weight loss over time.
  Typically treated with mesenteric bypass or transaortic endarterectomy where appropriate. Endovascular options exist and are used more and more.
- Acute mesenteric ischemia presents as "pain out of proportion to exam" that is sudden in onset. Diarrhea may be present, and exam may show hemodynamic instability as well as irregular heartbeat (depending on type of acute mesenteric ischemia). May also see distension, peritonitis, and blood per rectum.

- Three types of acute mesenteric ischemia: thrombotic, embolic, and non-occlusive.
  - NOMI (non-occlusive mesenteric ischemia)
    - Found in critically ill patients on vasopressors who demonstrate a low-flow condition
    - Mesenteric vessels are constricted
    - Treatment is NOT surgery. It is direct intra-arterial vasodilator therapy with papaverine and stopping vasopressors if possible.
    - Griffith's & Sudeck's may be affected.
    - Patients with this subtype have highest mortality risk (80-90%) versus overall 30-45% for all comers with acute mesenteric ischemia.
  - Embolic
    - SMA distal to middle colic artery is typically the level that is occluded
    - Proximal jejunum and transverse colon are typically spared.
    - First revascularize with embolectomy, bypass, etc. This allows marginal bowel to declare itself. Ressect dead bowel. Patient may need second look laparotomy for marginal areas. May use open abdomen technique.
  - Thrombotic
    - Typically seen at SMA origin where acute thrombosis forms at area of previous atherosclerosis.
    - Entire small intestine, right colon, and transverse colon are affected.
    - If proximal jejunum and transverse colon are spared, typically lesion is NOT thrombotic type.
    - Treatment is similar to embolic type: revascularize, resect, and second look for any areas that are questionable.
- Patients with hypercoagulable conditions/states most commonly thrombose the superior mesenteric vein. Treatment for venous occlusion includes anticoagulation with heparin followed by coumadinization. If peritonitis or ischemia develop due to this venous occlusion, patient requires laparotomy and resection.
- CT demonstrates lack of contrast flow, calcifications at origins of visceral arteries (celiac / SMA, etc.) along with findings of bowel ischemia such as stranding and wall thickening in acute mesenteric ischemia.

Visceral artery aneurysms

- Pancreatitis, portal HTN, and medial fibrodysplasia are risk factors among others
- All splanchnic artery aneurysm > 2cm when diagnosed must be repaired (EXCEPT for splenic artery aneurysms) because of 50% rupture rate.
- Splenic artery aneurysm is most common visceral aneurysm
  - Seen more commonly in women
  - 2% rupture risk
  - high rate of pregnancy related rupture (usually 3rd trimester)
  - repair if patient is pregnant, woman is of childbearing age, or is > 3-4 cm.
  - repair may include covered stent, bypass may be performed if that fails.
- If open procedure is performed, also may ligate splenic artery as alternative treatment because has good collaterals.

Renal artery aneurysm...Covered stent is treatment (perform if aneurysm > 1.5 cm)

Iliac artery aneurysm...If > 3.0 cm, covered stent

Femoral artery aneurysm...If > 2.5 cm, covered stent

Popliteal artery aneurysm

- Most common peripheral aneurysm
- ½ are bilateral (check both sides)
- ½ have another aneurysm elsewhere (check aorta)
- may get emboli or thrombosis with limb ischemia
- diagnosis based on ultrasound, and leg exam may demonstrate wide pulse at popliteal.
- if > 2 cm, symptomatic, or mycotic needs repair
- covered stent is NOT recommended for these
- Needs bypass and exclusion, otherwise 25% have complication that requires amputation if not treated

Renal artery stenosis

- 5% of hypertension patients have this
- Common cause of secondary hypertension
- Think of renal artery stenosis (RAS) in young patients with HTN that does not improve with medications or requires multiple medications.
- Also consider RAS in elderly patients with peripheral vascular disease (PVD).
- Causes include atherosclerosis, arterial dissection, Takayasu's, & re-stenosis post stenting.
- Another important cause is fibro-muscular dysplasia.
- Typically asymptomatic, and history demonstrates HTN that is NOT improved with multiple medications.
- Imaging demonstrates > 3.5 velocity ratio by duplex ultrasound when compared to aorta.
- "string of beads" sign seen on MRA or angio.
- Ratio of > 1.5 in renin levels between renal veins (one renal vein with elevated level compared to contralateral side) as sampled by catheter directed sampling is also diagnostic.
- ACE inhibitors actually worsen this condition and will accelerate renal failure. Some patients with RAS may be on these owing to initial attempts to control HTN.

Acute limb ischemia

- Embolic sources are afib, MI with mural thrombus, valvular vegetation, or a similar cardiac source in almost every case.
- Acute limb ischemia is a true surgical emergency.
- 6P's of limb ischemia include pain, pulselessness, parathesia, poikilothermia (cold), pallor and paralysis. (Often referred to as the 5Ps and paralysis is omitted from the mneumonic device.)
- Although pain is considered to be the most reliable indicator, a lack of pain does NOT rule out acute limb ischemia.
- Water-hammer pulse is palpable proximal to occlusion.
- May be thrombotic or embolic. Patients with thrombotic may report history of claudication that became worse.
- Diagnosis is typically made without imaging, but ultrasound may be useful.
- Empiric heparinization is indicated once this condition is suspected.
- Most patients should receive embolectomy, and a select few who are high risk and have a distal occlusion may be candidates for catheter directed therapy.
- Retrieved clot is typically sent to pathology to rule out atrial myxoma.
- Fasciotomy may be required depending upon ischemic time and surgeon judgment.
- Entire limb and proximal area should be prepped to allow for bypass revascularization if necessary.
- Angio is often used while in OR to demonstrate return of flow.
- Compartment syndrome may occur post operatively, and fasciotomy performed in the OR at initial case may be used to help prevent this. (See compartment syndrome under "Vascular injuries" section under Trauma chapter.)

Thoracic outlet syndrome

- Women more affected than men (except for cases of thoracic outlet syndrome that demonstrate venous compression)
- Symptoms typically seen in patient's 40s.
- Due to compression of neurovascular bundle as it exits thoracic cavity to innervate the arm. May be compressed by enlarged scalene muscle, cervical rib, repetitive motion injury, or neck trauma.
- Most common neurologic symptoms are pain and parasthesias.
- Holding arms over head or tilting head AWAY from the affected side will cause worsening of symptoms. Bruit at supraclavicular region may be present. Microemboli may be seen. EMG changes and hand muscle atrophy may be seen in extreme cases, but are unusual.
- Neck xrays can rule out rib compression or accessory rib. Young patients with occlusion of arteries in digits should receive angio with arm abducted and head in a neutral position.
- First rib resection may be required to treat. Cases caused by scalene musculature are typically treated with rest and physical therapy first.

Peripheral vascular disease

- Lower extremities are affected more often than upper.
- Typically caused by atherosclerosis.
- Five percent of patients older than 65 years of age will have symptomatic disease and 10% of that group will require amputation. Tobacco users and those with diabetes are more likely to require amputation.
- Patients typically present with claudication.
- Disease progresses from pain with exercise to pain at rest.
- Rest pain becomes tissue loss and ulceration if no treatment occurs.
- Leriche's syndrome is caused by aortoiliac disease and includes claudication of thigh, buttock, and calf. Impotence and diminished femoral pulses are seen.
- When pulses are diminished, obstruction is proximal to that level.
- Patients who have pallor of the extremity when elevated and rubor when in dependent position have significantly advanced arterial insufficiency. These physical exam findings help differentiate insufficiency from ischemia.
- Venous stasis disease gives an extremity that is purple in any position.
- Rest pain usually includes a burning type pain localized to the forefoot. Dangling the foot from the bed is an effort to use gravity to increase flow.
- Nonhealing wounds from minor trauma are seen. Little to know evidence of granulation is seen.
- Dry gangrene becomes wet gangrene with infection of the area.
- Although diagnosis is based on physical exam, noninvasive testing may be useful. Ankle SBP decreased greater than 20% after exercise is considered positive. Note that angio is the gold standard test.
- First steps in treatment are NON-invasive and include muscle conditioning (eg a walking program), risk factor reduction (blood glucose control and cholesterol control), and anti-platelet therapy (aspirin, clopidogrel, cilostazol, pentoxifylline).

- Rest pain, inability to maintain function, tissue necrosis and gangrene require intervention. May be endovascular or surgical.
- Open endarterectomy is typically NOT used for femoral endarterectomy owing to high restenosis rate.
- Fem-pop bypass is commonly used for disease limited to femoral / popliteal arteries. Saphenous vein, whether reversed or in-situ is preferred, but PTFE may be used to bypass to the above the knee popliteal artery. PTFE used beneath the knee has low patency rates and so is avoided.
- If bypass is distal to trifurcation, patency long term is low at approximately 50% and these are typically performed only for limb salvage.
- If large vessel has short segment disease, patient may be good candidate for endovascular repair. Endovascular repair is usually limited to such lesions.

Lower extremity ulcers and venous insufficiency

- More than 500,000 patients are affected yearly.
- Caused by failure / incompetency of valves in the deep venous system of the lower extremities.
- Varicose veins and edema result if no treatment is received.
- Hyperpigmentation and venous ulceration are additional sequelae.
- Duplex makes diagnosis of relux due to incompetent valves.
- Compression therapy with boots or stockings is the initial treatment along with wound care.
- Endoscopic perforator ligation or other surgical options exist when compression therapy and other initial therapies fail.

Lymphedema

- Typically a condition acquired from previous surgery / radiation therapy.
- Other potential causes include malignancy, filariasis, or primary lymphedema.
  Primary lymphedema includes lymphedema praecox, lymphedema tarda, and congenital lymphedema.
- Caused by disruption of lymphatics.
- Diagnosis is made by H&P.
- Hyperkeratoic skin, fluctuations in limb diameter, recurring cellulitis and skin weeping help make diagnosis.
- There is no cure. Treatments include elevation and compression. Lymphatic massage may reduce cellulitis recurrences.

Varicose veins

- Typical patient is an overweight female.
- Pain and fatigue in affected extremity are common symptoms. These symptoms worsen when legs are in dependent position.
- Compression stockings are initial treatment.
- Indications for surgical correction include failure of initial treatment and issues with cosmesis.
- Sclerotherapy, laser ablation, radiofrequency ablation, and saphenous vein striping are options for intervention.

Superficial thrombophlebitis

- Varicose veins or ones with current / previous catheters are more prone to be affected, but any vein may be affected.
- Physical exam makes diagnosis. Redness, warmth, tenderness to palpation & palpable cord may be present.
- Ultrasound is useful to determine whether any thrombus present extends into deep system.
- Suppurative thrombophlebitis (infected thrombophlebitis) is usually seen with indwelling catheters. May require excision.
- Superficial thrombophlebitis is usually treated with compression, heat, and anti-inflammatory meds.

Miscellaneous vascular diseases

- Fibromuscular dysplasia
  - Affects young women.
  - HTN may occur if renals are involved. Stroke or other neuro symptoms if carotids are involved.
  - Renal artery stenosis is seen and renals are most commonly involved vessels. Carotids second most common. Iliacs are third.
  - "string of beads" appearance on imaging.
  - Most common type is medial fibrodysplasia and this comprises 85% of cases.
  - PTA is considered best treatment, and bypass is performed if PTA fails.
- Cystic medial necrosis
  - Typically due to Marfan's disease. Marfan's is due to a fibrillin defect.
  - Marfanoid body habitus, aortic dilation and retinal issues such as detachment may be seen.
- Temporal arteritis
  - Most typically seen in women > 55.
  - Complaints may include headache, blindness, fever, headache, and blurred vision. Again, blindness may occur (!)
  - Biopsy of temporal artery may show giant cell arteritis and granulomas.
  - Inflammation of aorta and branches may also be seen.
  - Steroids are treatment. Bypass performed on larger vessels if steroids not effective.
- Raynaud's
  - Affects young women.
  - Typically color change seen on hands is white to blue to red. (Pallor to cyanosis to rubor.)
  - Calcium channel blockers are the treatment.

- Radiation enteritis
  - Thrombosis and sloughing of tissue is seen early owing to obliterative endarteritis.
  - Stenosis, scarring, and fibrosis is seen late (1-10 years)
  - Very advanced atherosclerosis may be seen 30 years later.
- Phlegmasia cerulea dolens
  - Painful, swollen blue leg owing to DVT. Particularly iliofemoral DVT.
  - More severe than albicans (next section).
  - May progress to gangrene.
  - Treatment is catheter directed thrombolysis, but emergent thrombectomy is indicated if threatened extremity.
  - Remember, about ½ of patients with this condition have malignancy elsewhere.
- Phlegmasia cerulea albicans
  Painful, swollen white lower extremity due to DVT. Less severe than dolens but may progress to dolens.

Select Subspecialties

Neurosurgery

- ADH release from posterior pituitary is controlled by supraoptic nucleus
  ADH increases water absorption in collecting ducts in response to increased osmolarity.
- Shock that may be seen in patients receiving radiotherapy for pituitary adenoma.
  - Diagnosis is pituitary apoplexy
  - Treatment is steroids.
- Blood supply to brain is from internal carotids (ICA) and vertebrals.
- ICA supplies hemispheres via anterior and middle cerebral arteries.
- Vertebrals supply portion of hemispheres as well as cerebellum and brainstem via (ultimately) posterior cerebral artery and basilar arteries.
- The anasatamosis between the branches of the ICA and vertebrals is the Circle of Willis.
- Artery of Adamkiewicz supplies conus medullaris and inferior portion of thoracic cord. Originates at T10-L2 area.
- Brain tumors
  - In adults, 2/3 of brain tumors are supratentorial. In children, 2/3 of brain tumors are infratentorial
  - Pituitary adenoma is treated with bromocriptine and trans-sphenoidal resection. Acromegaly, loss of peripheral vision, and galactorrhea may be seen.
  - Medulloblastoma: Increased ICP and cerebellar dysfunction are seen. Most common primary brain tumor in children. (Most common metastatic brain tumor in children is neuroblastoma.) Radiation, chemotherapy, and resection are treatments.
  - Ependymoma: If seen in childhood, lesion is most commonly seen in posterior fossa. In adults, supratentorial position. Involves central canal or 4th ventricle, so increased ICP is seen and hydrocephalus. Resection is treatment. Radiation may be used as an adjunct
  - Acoustic neuroma: Treatment is resection. This is a schwannoma. Tinnitus, one sided hearing loss, vertigo, hydrocephalus maybe seen. Neurofibromatosis association
  - Meningioma : Approximately 20% of intra-cranial tumors . Most commonly seen in middle aged women . Unilateral proptosis, inability to perceive smell, and calcifications are seen . While prognosis is excellent if completely resected, lack of complete resection give high risk for recurrence.
  - Oligodendroglioma: Classic history is patient with long history of seizures . Slow growing tumor that affects young / middle aged patients. Common in children. Chemoradiation and resection.
  - Glioblastoma multiforme: Gliomas are most common type of primary brain tumor. Glioblastoma multiforme is most common type of glioma seen. Actually a grade 4 astrocytoma . Represents ¼ of primary brain tumor cases, which is unfortunate because average survival is 11 months . Presents with bleeding, focal neurologic deficits, increased ICP . Radiation, chemo, and resection if possible. Steroid dosing (eg dexamethasone) to control edema.

- Astrocytoma: High grade lesions are seen in older patients, low grade lesions in younger patients. Resection (if possible), chemo, and radiation. Unfortunately, most degenerate into glioblastoma multiforme with time.

- Arteriovenous malformations
  - Congenital, but symptoms commonly do not arise until 20-40 YOA
  - Bleeding or sudden intense headache is presentation
  - Seizures, loss of consciousness, or neck stiffness may also be presentation
  - Non-contrast head CT makes diagnosis
  - HTN control, Ca++ channel blockers (to prevent vasospasms), and radiotherapy or embolization are treatment
- Brown Sequard syndrome: one side of cord is transected. Same side as injury loses motor function and other functions. Opposite side loses ability to feel pain, temperature, and light touch.
- Central cord syndrome
  - From either bleeding into central portion of cord, infarct of central portion of cord, or (more commonly) hyper-extension. Upper extremities become weak, and patches of skin become hyper-esthetic (very sensitive) while others lose sensation.
  - May be seen in elderly trauma patients who do NOT have neck fractures. (From hyperextension with pre-existing arthritic changes.)
  - May NOT be present with symptoms in trauma bay, but may emerge later.
- Anterior cord syndrome
  - Loss of blood supply to anterior portion of cord.
  - Results in inability to move bilaterally and loss of pain and temp sensation bilaterally.
- Spine tumor facts
  - Most common spine tumor is neurofibroma
  - Most spine tumors are benign.
  - Extradural tumors are more commonly malignant while intradural tumors are more commonly benign.
  - For paraganglionomas, remember to check urine metanephrines.
- Broca's area: infarct gives broken speech. Located at posterior part of anterior lobe. ("Broca's gives Broken speech.")
- Wernicke's area: temporal lobe location, speech comprehension.

OB/Gyn

- Uterine artery and ovarian artery provide blood supply to ovary
- At squamocolumnar junction, cervix goes from stratified squamous epithelium to columnar epithelium. This location is the most common site for cervical cancer.
- 28 day menstrual cycles is divided into follicular, ovulatory, and luteal phases.
- Follicle stimulating hormone (FSH) and lutenizing hormone (LH) released from pituitary. This oocyte to mature. FSH is then inhibited by increasing estrogen levels. A dominant follicle continues through the cycle and produces estrogen.
- Approximately 14 days into the cycle, estrogen and LH increase. This results in the ovary releasing the dominant follicle and the egg enters the fallopian tube. Cervix is prepared for sperm via thickening and increasing levels of mucous.
- Corpus luteum formed from empty follicle. Corpus luteum secretes estrogen and progesterone. Fertilization may take place.
- Endometriosis
    - Affects 20% of women of reproductive age
    - Infertility may occur
    - Retrograde menstruation is one potential cause, but cause is generally unknown
    - Most commonly found in locations outside uterus
    - Pelvic pain, infertility, menorrhagia, pelvic mass, nodular uterosacral ligament—all may be present
    - MRI or ultrasound may be consistent with diagnosis, but exploratory laparotomy is confirmatory.
    - Lesions are blue and black. May appear similar to "gunpowder burns" or "chocolate cysts".
    - Treatment is NSAIDs for pain, oral contraceptive pills, danazol, an GnRH agonists.
    - Surgery may be utilized to improve fertility and anatomic relationships.

- Gynecologic conditions that may cause acute abdomen
    - Ovarian torsion
    - Ectopic pregnancy (ruptured or otherwise)
    - Pelvic Inflammatory Disease (PID)
- Endometrial cancer
    - This is the most common malignancy of the reproductive tract in the female
    - Adenocarcinoma is most common
    - Tamoxifen use, diabetes, obesity, polycystic ovarian syndrome, hypertension are all risk factors.
    - Postmenopausal vaginal bleeding is most common presentation
    - Diagnosis is made with endometrial biopsy.
    - Radiotherapy may be used if nodes are positive or high grade lesion
- Ovarian lesions (cysts and cancer)
    - Age > 50 is associated with increased risk of malignant ovarian lesion
    - A solid, fixed pelvic mass in a peri or post menopausal woman is consistent with ovarian cancer
    - Meige's syndrome is ovarian fibroma that causes hydrothorax and ascites
    - Lesion removal is curative.
    - Metastatic lesions of the ovary are called Krunkenberg tumors (may be from any site, but classic is from GI tract)
    - Most common metastatic GI lesion to the ovary is gastric cancer
    - CA-125 helps differentiate malignant lesions from benign lesions.

- Often laparotomy is necessary to determine whether a cystic ovarian lesion is benign or malignant without laparotomy and pathology review.
    - Malignant ovarian lesions
        - Serous cystadenoma
            - May be bilateral
            - Fluid filled lesion with tall columnar epithelium
        - Mucinous cystadenoma
            - Mucin production
            - Similar to intestinal or endocervical epithelium
        - Sertoli-leydig tumor
          Results in excess testosterone and virilization
        - Granulosa-thecal cell tumor
          Results in precocious puberty
        - Choriocarcinoma
          Most frequently seen after a molar pregnancy. Increased HCG is seen. Treated with chemo or total abdominal hysterectomy.
        - Teratoma (immature)
            - Seen in young females
            - Increased AFP is seen.
            - In mature teratomas, adult tissue such as hair and teeth are seen. These are not seen in immature teratomas.
        - Dysgerminoma
            - Most common germ cell ovarian tumor that is malignant
            - Seen in second to third decade of life
            - Increased CA 125, increased LDH.
            - Is sensitive to both radiation and chemotherapy

- Cervical cancer
    - Second most common cancer of reproductive system in female
    - Typically seen in women 45-55 years old
    - Most commonly is squamous cell carcinoma at the transition zone
    - Risk factors are HPV 16, 18, and 31 as well as early sexual activity, multiple partners, chronic cervical inflammation and tobacco use
    - Painless post-coital vaginal bleeding is the classic symptom
    - Pap smear is only 50% sensitive, and colposcopy with biopsy is required for suspicious areas
    - A loop electrical excisional procedure (LEEP) with conization should be performed when moderate or severe dysplasia is present.

- Treatment of cervical cancer by stage
  - FIGO Stage 1: carcinoma at cervix
  - Stage 2: spread to upper two thirds of vagina, parametrial involvement may be present
  - Stage 3: lower one third of vagina involved or pelvic wall involvement
  - Stage 4: bladder involved, rectum involved, or + distant metastasis
  - Carcinoma in situ and stage 1: remove transition zone via cryotherapy, laser treatment, cone biopsy or LEEP. Hyseterectomy is an option is patient does not want fertility in the future.
  - Stage 1A2, 1B, or 2: radical hysterectomy, pelvic node dissection
  - Other stages: radiation (internal or external)
- Vulvar and vaginal cancer
  - Most common SCC associated with HPV.
  - Diethylstilbestrol (DES) exposure gives increased risk for vaginal clear cell carcinoma
  - Vaginal bleeding, itching, and discharge may be present.
  - May be treated with vaginectomy with or without radiation.
  - Wide local excision is acceptable for vulvar cancer with microinvasion, but radical vulvectomy with node dissection is required for more advanced lesions.

Urology

- Gerota's fascia envelops the kidneys. They are retroperitoneal organs.
- Anatomy including renal vein length and position was discussed in earlier section. Renal vein on L is longer than R. On L, gonadal vein drains into renal vein.
- Kidney functions
  - Regulates RBC production via erythropoietin
  - Regulates blood pressure
    - Juxtaglomerular apparatus regulates according to renal blood flow (both osmolarity and pressure).
    - Renin release is increased in response to low BP or decreased osmolarity. Aldosterone increases as a result, and sodium resorption occurs.
  - Regulates vitamin D production
    1,25 dihydroxycholecalciferol (vitamin D active form) is in part made in the kidneys
  - Excretes waste
  - Regulates H20 and electrolytes
    Regulation of water at the collecting ducts is regulated by ADH (vasopressin), while Na+ reabsorption is controlled by aldosterone.
- Remember to rule out an intra-abdominal condition when patient has an isolated L sided varicocele because L gonadal vein drains into L renal vein.
- In men (unlike women) an internal and external sphincter controls urinary continence and ejaculation
- The prostate creates seminal fluid via seminal vesicles.
- Sertoli cells are responsible for spermatogenesis.
- Leydig cells make testosterone.

- Sperm follows the SEVU path: seminal vesicles, epididymis, vas deferens, urethra.
- Note that the ejaculatory duct is formed from the seminal vesicles and vas deferens.
- Remember at renal hilum it's VAN: renal Vein, renal Artery, and Ureter from anterior to posterior.
- Renal angiotensin aldosterone system: decreased osmolarity gives increased renin. This causes cleavage of angiotensinogen to angiotensin 1. Angiotensin 1 is then converted to angiotensin 2 via angiotensin converting enzyme in the lungs. This results in increased aldosterone.
- Testicular tumors
    - Most common cancer in men 20-35 years
    - Cryptorchidism is a risk factor and increases risk for both testicles
    - Solid, firm, painless testicular mass is typical presentation
    - Testicular ultrasound confirms diagnosis
    - CT abdomen and pelvis along with CXR evaluates for metastatic disease.
    - Radical orchiectomy via inguinal approach makes definitive diagnosis and is portion of treatment.
    - Seminomas are highly radiosensitive.
- Nephrolithiasis
    - Typically seen in males 20-50 years old.
    - Presents as colicky flank pain and hematuria.
    - 90% of stones are radio-opaque and so are visible on KUB
    - non-contrast abdominal CT is the preferred diagnostic imaging study
    - conservative management includes pain control and hydration.
    - Stones less than 5mm in size will usually pass spontaneously
    - Extra-corporeal shock wave lithotripsy may be used for non-obstructing stones less than 3cm in size
    - Larger stones often require percutaneous nephrolithotomy
    - Nephrolithiasis by type
        - Struvite stone: Caused by bacteria (such as proteus mirabilis) that produce urease. Associated with UTIs. Staghorn appearance to calculi. Treated with hydration and antibiotics for UTI treatment.
        - Calcium oxalate: Radio-opaque. Treat with hydration.
        - Uric acid: Found in conditions associated with high purine (DNA bases adenine and guanine) turnover. Also associated with conditions with high uric acid levels (eg gout. These are radiolucent. Treat with hydration and urine alkalinization.
        - Cysteine: Caused by cysteine transport defect. Radio-opaque. Treat with hydration and urine alkalinization.

- Renal cell carcinoma
    - Most typically seen in men during sixth decade of life
    - 95% of renal neoplasms
    - risk factors include family history of renal cancer, syndromes associated with renal cancer, and tobacco use.
    - Classic triad of flank pain, hematuria (mico or macroscopic), and palpable mass may be present.
    - Paraneoplastic conditions such as hypercalcemia, polycythemia, cushing's syndrome, bone pain, or HTN may be present.
    - Renal ultrasound or abdominal CT confirms diagnosis. Commonly a vascularized, solid mass will be visualized.
    - CXR and bone scan assess for distant disease.
    - Remember, lesion may also be metastatic from lung, breast, stomach, contralateral kidney or another site.
    - Nephrectomy, chemo, radio, immuno and hormonal therapy all play a role in treatment.
    - Survival for stage 4 disease is < 20% but for stage 1 disease is 94%.
        - Stage 1 = < 7cm, limited to kidney, nodes not involved
        - Stage 2 = > 7cm, limited to kidney, nodes not involved.
        - Stage 3 = any sized tumor limited to kidney with 1 or more nodes involved, or any sized tumor that invades nearby structure.
        - Stage 4 = any tumor that invades beyond Gerota's fascia that involves > 1 regional node or any tumor that has distant metastases present.

- Prostate cancer
  - Most common cancer in men
  - 2nd most common cause of death due to cancer in men
  - most commonly seen in men in 8th decade
  - most frequently is an adenocarcinoma
  - Risk factors include increased age, family history of cancer, African American race, and high dietary fat.
  - Often asymptomatic, and may be discovered incidentally during digital rectal exam.
  - May present as bone pain, lower extremity edema, urinary obstruction, or lower extremity edema (among other ways).
  - PSA will be increased.
  - Transrectal ultrasound guided biopsy is required to confirm diagnosis.
  - CXR and bone scan are used to evaluate for metastatic disease.
  - Multiple treatment options exist, including observation, radiation therapy, radical prostatectomy, androgen deprivation (flutamide) or a combination of options.
  - Prostatectomy complications include impotence and incontinence.
  - Stage 1 five year survival is approximately 100%, and five year survival for stage 4 disease is approximately 30%
    - Stage 1 = tumor that is incidentally discovered, nodes negative
    - Stage 2 = palpable disease that is confined to prostate, nodes negative.
    - Stage 3 = disease beyond prostate capsule, invasion may or may not be present into seminal vesicles, nodes negative
    - Stage 4 = disease invades adjacent structures (other than seminal vesicles), or present in nodes or distant locations.

- Urinary incontinence
  - Approximately 13 million patients in US are affected
  - Risk factors: UTI, childbirth, medications, BPH, birth defects, spinal cord abnormality, neuropathy, pelvic floor / bladder weakness, and prolapse.
  - Types
    - Urge
      - Overactivity of detrusor muscle.
      - Patient feels need to void and has inability to prevent voiding.
    - Stress

      Intra-abdominal pressure exceeds the pressure of urethral sphincter (eg coughing produces leakage)

    - Overflow

      Ongoing inability to fully empty bladder. Due to urethral obstruction or spinal cord abnormalities

    - Mixed
    - Combination of above types
  - Diagnosis is clinical, and urodynamic tests allow clarification of which type is present.
  - Kegel exercises, lifestyle changes (tobacco cessation, antihistamines, avoiding diuretics), medications (eg oxybutynin, doxazosin, tamsulosin), TURP (for BPH induced overflow incontinence) may be utilized.
  - In particular, stress incontinence may be amenable to urethropexy or suburethral sling.
  - Urge incontinence may be treated with bladder augmentation.

- Bladder cancer
  - Typically transitional cell cancer
  - Most commonly affects men in 7th decade
  - Tobacco use, increased age, and chemical exposure (eg aniline dye, benzidine, cyclophosphamide, phenacetin) are typical risk factors.
  - Chronic inflammation (from a condition such as schistosomiasis) is an additional risk factor.
  - Schistosomiasis is associated with squamous cell cancer (of the bladder).
  - Symptoms include micro or macroscopic hematuria
  - Cystoscopy with biopsy makes diagnosis
  - Superficial tumors may be treated with transurethral resection and intravesicular chemo (BCG vaccine or doxorubicin)
  - For invasive cancers which are localized, radical cystectomy with urinary diversion is treatment.
  - Advanced bladder cancer is treated with a cisplatin based regimen.

Otolaryngology

- Sternocleidomastoid divides neck into anterior and posterior triangles
    - Anterior triangle
        - Arteries present include facial, internal carotid and external carotid
        - Major nerves include glossopharyngeal (cranial nerve 9), vagus (CN 10), hypoglossal (CN 12)
        - Veins present include facial vein, anterior jugular and internal jugular
        - Lymph node groups include submental and submandibular
        - Glands present are submandibular, parotid and thyroid
        - Muscles include SCM, suprahyoid, digastric and infrahyoid
    - Posterior triangle
        - Artery present is subclavian artery
        - Nerve present is spinal accessory nerve (CN 11)
        - Veins present are external jugular and subclavian vein
        - Lymph node group is cervical nodes
        - No major named glands are present
        - Muscles include SCM, trapezius, splenius capitus, levator scapulae, and anterior & posterior scalene

- Salivary gland tumor facts

  - Commonly present as painless masses, but at times pain may be present.
  - Facial paralysis associated with nerve invasion may be seen. Nerve invasion is worrisome for malignancy.
  - Types
    - Pleiomorphic adenoma is most common benign tumor
      - Tends to affect males
      - tends to be bilateral
      - Warthin's tumor is 2nd most common benign tumor
    - Mucoepidermoid is most common malignant tumor
    - Adenoid cystic is second most common malignant salivary tumor, except in minor salivary glands where it is the most common malignant salivary tumor
    - Most common childhood salivary tumor is hemangioma
  - FNA of mass or involved node is used to determine whether benign or malignant.
  - CT demonstrates node status.
  - Size is determining factor for staging.
    - T1 is < 2cm, T2 is between T1 and T3, and T3 is > 4cm.
  - Benign parotid tumors are treated with superficial parotidectomy.
  - Malignant salivary lesions are treated with resection of gland from which tumor originates, modified radical neck dissection, and at times post op radiation with exceptions as noted in next bullet point. Radiation is used if recurrent disease, margins are positive, T3 or greater disease, or invasion of surrounding structures.
  - Malignancies that are < 4cm, low grade, and located in superifical lobe of parotid may be treated with superficial parotidectomy.

- Complications of resection include nerve injuries to cranial nerve 12, cranial nerve 7 (mandibular branch), the greater auricular nerve, and the auriculotemporal nerve. Damage to auriculotemporal nerve may result in Frey's syndrome, which is sweating while eating ("gustatory sweating") owing to abnormal innervation of parasympathetic fibers.
- Modified radical neck dissection preserves CN 11, sternocleidomastoid, and the internal jugular vein.
- There is an approximately 15% risk of second primary head and neck tumor when a first primary tumor is discovered.

- Oral tumors
  - Most (90%) are squamous cell carcinomas.
  - Most typical location is tongue of male patient
  - Erythroplakia (red patch) or leukoplakia (white patch) are premalignant antecedents of cancer.
  - Painless mass or ulcer that may be associated with bleeding, pain, and speech changes.
  - Imaging (CT and MRI) are used to determine lesion relationship to other structures and size.
  - Laryngoscopy with biopsy gives diagnosis.
  - TNM staging
    - T1 <2cm, T2 is between T1 and T3, T3 is > 4cm, T4 is tumor invades surrounding structures (a=resectable tumor, b=not resectable)
    - N0 is negative regional nodes. N1 is positive ipsilateral node < or equal to 3cm, N2 is one or multiple nodes positive > 3cm or < 6cm, N3 is lymph node(s) greater than 6cm
    - M0 is no metastatic disease, M1 is positive metastatic disease.
  - Size is major determining factor for staging
    - T1 is < 2cm, T2 is between T1 and T3, and T3 is > 4cm.
    - Stage 1 is T1N0M0
Stage 2 is T2N0M0
Stage 3 is T3N0M0 or T1-3N1M0
Stage 4a is T4aN0/N1M0 or T1-4aN2M0
Stage 4b is Any T, N3M0 or T4b, any N, M0
Stage 4c is Any T any N M1
Five year survival is approximately 80% for T1 disease to approximately 20% for T4 disease.

- Laryngeal cancer
  - Most commonly men in 5th to 7th decade
  - Risk factors include tobacco and alcohol use.
  - Presents as hoarseness, painful swallowing, or airway obstruction
  - Tracheostomy is typically required to secure airway.
  - Tumor location and vocal cord function determine treatment. May include radiation, chemoradiation, and / or surgery.
  - Modified radical neck dissection is used if nodes are involved.
  - Survival is 95% with stage 1 disease but 20% with stage 4 disease.
- Retropharyngeal abscess
  - Anaerobic, aerobic, or gram negative bacteria may be causal.
  - Seen in children and adults.
  - Drooling, irritability, still neck, an airway obstruction may occur.
  - Airway obstruction due to retropharyngeal abscess is "Ludwig's angina".
  - Posterior pharyngeal bulge may be seen and patient may hold neck toward UNAFFECTED side.
  - Pharyngeal widening is seen on neck xray.
  - First secure the airway, and only THEN explore the lesion, drain, and give antibiotics.
  - Mediastinitis may occur and carries a 50% mortality.
  - Aspiration, pneumonia, empyema and death can occur,

- Peritonsillar abscess
  - Gives "hot potato" voice
  - Commonly a polymicrobial infection
  - Empiric coverage for streptococcus is required.
  - Seen in young adults
  - Uvula deviates toward contralateral side
  - Anterior tonsillar pillar bulges
  - Needle aspiration will be diagnostic and therapeutic, but exam will usually confirm diagnosis before aspiration.
  - If aspiration fails, may require incision and drainage.

How To Unlock Your Video Review Course

More than five hundred and fifty hours of work went in to making this review book and the online course!

Like this promo shares, unlike every other ABSITE review book available, this one comes with that video review course presented by the author of *ABSITE Smackdown!* No need for a plane ticket to another city or a $595 fee (that's the price of other ABSITE review courses) because your course is all included.

And here's how you unlock that course for you to use anytime and anywhere on your computer, phone, or tablet.

It's easy and only takes one email!

You may have purchased the book as a paperback or on one of the online platforms like Amazon, Shopify, or Podio.

Wherever you bought it, just forward your receipt via email to

info@TheHealthcareLab.org

and that's it! Usually the team will reply within 24 hours with a coupon code and link to the online course. That code will unlock your course access.

Notice that the address ends with .org and NOT .com!

The Healthcare Lab, Inc. will NOT share your email address with any third party.

The team is excited to share the video review course, which follows the content in the book, and looks forward to hearing from you!

About The Author

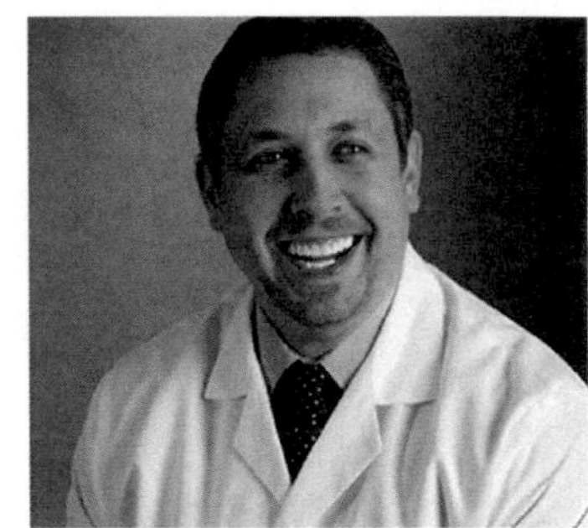

DAVID KASHMER is a quality improvement expert, & trauma and acute-care surgeon.

He earned his Medical Doctorate degree from MCP Hahnemann University--now Drexel University College of Medicine--and his Bachelor of Science degree in Biology from Villanova University through a joint BS-MD program with MCP Hahnemann.

He has previously served as a Section Chief, Chief of Surgery, & Chief Medical Officer for healthcare organizations. He currently serves as a general surgery residency program director.

David also earned a Lean Six Sigma Master Black Belt certificate at Villanova. Dr. Kashmer holds a Master of Business Administration degree in Healthcare Administration from George Washington University. He previously served on the Board of Examiners for the Malcolm Baldrige National Quality Award.

David has authored multiple books on healthcare quality improvement including several Amazon Bestsellers.

One Last Thing...

A note from The Healthcare Lab, Inc. team:

If this book was useful to you or if you enjoyed it, we'd really appreciate your review on Amazon.

The support is very important and we do read each and every review so that this work can be updated and improved.

If you're reading the paperback version of the book, we'd appreciate your comments on Amazon.com.

If you're reading this on Kindle, Amazon will ask you for a review. (In just a moment.)

If you've picked up *ABSITE Smackdown!* on any other platform, please drop a review if you liked the work.

If you enjoyed the book, please take a moment and pass along your feedback!

One great way to do that is to type this link on your computer, phone, or tablet and tell us directly about what you think:

http://bit.ly/ABSITESmackdownFeedback

Other Books From The Healthcare Lab, Inc.

Ten Secrets: A Healthcare Quality Improvement Handbook

Use these Ten Secrets from the quality experts to make your next quality improvement project great!

Ten secrets, six experts, and over 50 years of combined healthcare quality improvement experience means zero problems for you and your team.

If 99.9% correct were ok in high-stakes fields, it would be fine if a plane crash happened just about every day at a busy airport like Boston's Logan, Philadelphia International, or Tampa International Airport. After all, people would say, 99.9% is good enough, right?

In fact, 99.9% error-free is not ok in Healthcare. And in *Ten Secrets*, national quality experts including Malcom Baldrige Award reviewers, Lean Six Sigma Master Black Belts, and practicing healthcare providers share key, high-level information to help get you and your team beyond routine levels of performance...because the patients are worth it.

Games for Health: Ultimate Beginner's Guide To Using Game Dynamics In Healthcare Organizations

Let's make working in healthcare even more fun...and effective!

There's an engagement crisis among healthcare workers...

According to recent reports, 70% of workers are either not engaged in their work or are actively trying to hurt their company. This lack of engagement leads to missed opportunities, revenue problems, and quality issues. One useful solution is the application of game dynamics to your current system and culture--and this work provides the tools to do just that. Use *Games for Health* to apply game dynamics to healthcare settings in order to facilitate culture change, quality improvement, and better patient care!

Trauma Program Operator's Manual

The Practical, Insider's Guide To Running A Trauma Program

The Trauma Program Operator's Manual Gives You Tools To Succeed!

If you're involved with a trauma program in any way, this manual is for you. It's filled with useful, hard to find info that helps guide your trauma program to excellence and beyond!

Healthcare Information System Hacking: Protect Your System

Understand how your health information is at risk and how hackers attempt to obtain it.

Healthcare Information System Hacking tells you specifics about what you need to protect your private health information, whether you're a system administrator, patient, or healthcare provider.

Learn the true value of your health information, and how hackers attempt to access it. *Healthcare Information System Hacking* introduces the specific steps hackers follow to obtain information from a hospital or health system. This book is great for information professionals in healthcare and concerned patients alike!

Made in the
USA
Middletown, DE